Hepatitis - Recent Advances in 2025

Edited by Xingshun Qi and Chengwei Tang

Published in London, United Kingdom

Hepatitis - Recent Advances in 2025
http://dx.doi.org/10.5772/intechopen.111136
Edited by Xingshun Qi and Chengwei Tang

Contributors
Alma Trnačević, Asma Mahdi, Azra Gutić Hodžić, Chengwei Tang, Cătălin Ştefan Ghenea, Danijel Bijedić, Dilista Piljić, Dokmeci Abdulkadir, Haonan Zhao, Harputluoglu Murat, Humera Porobić-Jahić, Jasminka Petrović, Jiafeng Ge, Livia Marieta Negoiţă, Mariana Mihăilă, Nagham Nafiz Hendi, Naiera M. Helmy, Pengpeng Xie, Rahima Jahić, Randa AlYafie, Sergey Netesov, Victor Manuylov, Xingshun Qi

First published in London, United Kingdom, 2025 by IntechOpen
IntechOpen is the global imprint of INTECHOPEN LIMITED, registered in England and Wales, registration number: 11086078, 167-169 Great Portland Street, London, W1W 5PF, United Kingdom

For EU product safety concerns: IN TECH d.o.o., Prolaz Marije Krucifikse Kozulić 3, 51000 Rijeka, Croatia, info@intechopen.com or visit our website at intechopen.com.

British Library Cataloguing-in-Publication Data
A catalogue record for this book is available from the British Library

Hepatitis - Recent Advances in 2025
Edited by Xingshun Qi and Chengwei Tang
p. cm.
Print ISBN 978-1-83634-341-7
Online ISBN 978-1-83634-340-0
eBook (PDF) ISBN 978-1-83634-342-4

Meet the editors

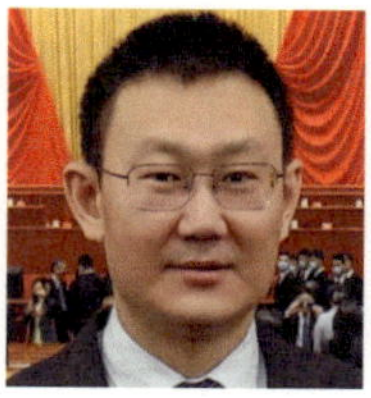

Dr. Xingshun Qi is the Head of the Department of Gastroenterology of the General Hospital of Northern Theater Command, China. His primary research interests are in clinical research related to the etiology, diagnosis, and management of liver cirrhosis, portal hypertension, portal vein thrombosis, Budd-Chiari syndrome, and hepatocellular carcinoma. He serves as a senior editorial board member of *BMC Gastroenterology*, an editorial board member of *Advances in Therapy and Therapeutic Advances in Gastroenterology,* and an academic editor of the *Canadian Journal of Gastroenterology and Hepatology* and the *Journal of Clinical and Translational Hepatology*. His H-index is 53 now.

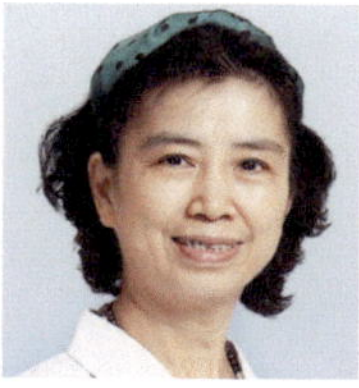

Prof. Dr. Chengwei Tang is the Director of the Department of Gastroenterology of the West China Hospital of Sichuan University, China. Her main research interests include liver cirrhosis with portal hypertension, acute pancreatitis, intestinal mucosal immunity, gastrointestinal polypeptides, and medical education. Currently, she serves as the President of the Chinese Society of Gastroenterology, Vice President of the Gastroenterology Physician Branch of the Chinese Medical Doctor Association, Executive Member of the Council of the Asian Pacific Association of Gastroenterology, and Deputy Chief Editor of the nationally planned textbook "Internal Medicine". She has been honored as a National Advanced Medical Worker and a Renowned National Doctor, and has won the first prize in the First National Textbook Construction Award, among other accolades.

Contents

Preface

Nowadays, viral hepatitis remains a major threat to public health with high prevalence and mortality worldwide, despite its significant decrease by the use of highly effective antivirals and the implementation of universal vaccination programs The WHO has launched an important initiative to reduce the number of new hepatitis infections by 90% and the number of deaths by 65% between 2016 and 2030. The physicians and scientists are striving to achieve this goal. Meanwhile, we have witnessed an increasing number of innovative findings regarding hepatitis.

In this setting, the book project *Hepatitis – Recent Advances in 2025*, published by IntechOpen, aims to collect chapters that summarize recent advances in the field of viral hepatitis. Finally, a total of six chapters have been accepted and compiled in the current book, which is divided into two major sections. In the first section regarding epidemiology of hepatitis B virus infection, one chapter by the researchers from Romania reviews the epidemiology of hepatitis B virus infection worldwide, transmission, prevention, genotype, and co-infection, and another chapter by the researchers from Russia systematically analyzed the HBsAg prevalence in the conditionally healthy population of Russia in 1982–2023. In the second section regarding management of hepatitis, one chapter by the researchers from Egypt illustrated the relationship between the microbiome and the hepatitis C virus, one chapter by the researchers from Bosnia and Herzegovina reported the experiences regarding diagnosis and treatment of a case with severe acute hepatitis B virus infection, one chapter written by us from China reviews the status quo about the management of chronic hepatitis B virus infection. Another chapter by the researchers from Jordan and Qatar introduces the advantage of precision medicine in managing viral hepatitis.

Herein, we would like to thank the authors worldwide for their significant contributions to completing their chapters, as well as the assistance from Karmen Daleta, a Publishing Process Manager at IntechOpen, in editing this book project. Dr. Xingshun Qi is also very indebted to the support from his family and study group. Finally, we hope that this book project is meaningful for clinicians, researchers, and patients in understanding the current knowledge about anticoagulation.

Dr. Xingshun Qi
Department of Gastroenterology,
General Hospital of Northern Theater Command,
Shenyang, China

Chengwei Tang
Professor,
Department of Gastroenterology,
West China Hospital,
Sichuan University,
Chengdu, China

Section 1

Hepatitis B

Chapter 1

Epidemiology of Hepatitis B Virus Infection

Mariana Mihăilă, Cătălin Ştefan Ghenea and Livia Marieta Negoiță

Abstract

Hepatitis B virus infection is one of the most common infectious pathologies spread globally, the prevalence being differently distributed from a geographical point of view. There are an estimated 350 million people infected with hepatitis B virus (HBV), the prevalence being high (>8%), intermediate (2–7%) and low (<2%). Approximately 1/3 of the world's population has an HBV exposure marker, characterized by the presence of HBc antibodies in the serum. In the last two decades, the number of cases of acute or chronic HBV infection has decreased due to the anti-HBV vaccination programs, the increase in the socioeconomic level and the access to antiviral treatment. In the absence of specific measures, the number of deaths due to the evolution of chronic HBV infection (liver cirrhosis, hepatocarcinoma, liver failure) is predicted to reach 1.14 million in 2035. In this chapter, we discuss the main ways of transmission of the hepatitis B virus along with effective prevention strategies.

Keywords: hepatitis B virus, epidemiology, prevention, hepatocarcinoma, liver failure

1. Introduction

Hepatitis B virus (HBV) infection is one of the most common infectious pathologies spread globally and is an important cause of acute and chronic liver disease, particularly in developing countries [1]. According to the World Health Organization (WHO), nearly 300 million people are chronically infected with HBV globally, with 1.5 million new infections each year. In 2019, hepatitis B resulted in an estimated 820,000 deaths, mostly from decompensated cirrhosis and hepatocellular carcinoma (HCC); as a result, HBV infection was ranked 15th among all causes of human mortality [2]. There are regional variations in the prevalence of chronic HBV infection: 0.1–2.0% in Western Europe and the United States, 2.0–8.0% in Japan and the Mediterranean region, and 8.0–20.0% in Southeast Asia and Sub-Saharan Africa [3].

A significant public health concern in the majority of nations is hepatitis B virus (HBV) infection, with an estimated 2 billion persons globally expressing viral exposure, and 360 million people have a chronic infection that is susceptible to liver disorders caused by HBV [4]. The hepatitis B virus (HBV) is responsible for acute and chronic hepatitis, cirrhosis, liver failure, and hepatocellular carcinoma (HCC) [5].

Significant death rates from this malignancy (HCC) are found in regions with a high endemicity of chronic HBV infection [6].

It represents the sixth most prevalent type of cancer worldwide and the third leading cause of cancer-related deaths [7]. Hepatitis B virus was initially named as serum hepatitis to differentiate it from hepatitis A virus, which was responsible for fecal-oral hepatitis [8]. HBV is the common form of viral hepatitis with parenteral transmission that causes acute and chronic hepatitis, some with progression to liver failure [9].

The clinical manifestations of acute infection resemble those of other viral hepatitis, and the incubation period varies between 1 and 6 months [10]. HBV hepatitis becomes chronic more frequently when the virus is contracted at a young age, 90% of infected infants and up to 30% of children. The later the infection is contracted, during adulthood, the risk of chronicity decreases to 5–10%, most having a complete recovery but with a serological scar, meaning the presence of anti-HBc antibodies in the blood [11]. Fulminant hepatitis occurs in rare cases, less than 1% of cases, and especially in immunocompromised people [12].

2. Transmission

In terms of the way the virus is transmitted, there is vertical transmission (perinatal) and horizontal transmission (**Table 1**) [13]. The first category appears during childbirth, from infected mothers who transmit it to their children [13]. The second way is horizontal transmission, which is divided into sexual and parenteral transmission through skin continuity solutions, blood transfusions, nosocomial infections, drug injections, and tattoos [14]. The development of chronic hepatitis B virus infection depends on how the virus spreads, as the risk decreases with age at infection for susceptible individuals [9].

HBV infection is transmitted through contact with infected body fluids, and it is only natural host is humans [15]. Blood is the most important vehicle of transmission, but other body fluids have also been implicated, including semen and saliva [16].

Perinatal transmission	• Infected mothers to neonates around birth (the babies born to HBeAg-positive mothers are particularly at risk. Approximately 90% of these kids continue to be chronically infected)
Sexual transmission	• Men who had sex with men • Promiscuous heterosexual (the length of sexual activity, the number of partners, the history of sexually transmitted disease, and a positive syphilis serology are all linked to an elevated risk of HBV infection in heterosexuals) • Sexual partners of injectable drug users • Prostitutes, and clients of prostitutes
Parenteral/ percutaneous	• Transfusion of blood products • Contaminated equipment used for therapeutic injections • Healthcare-related procedures (e.g., patients on a hemodialysis program) • needle sharing by intravenous drug users • piercing or tattooing

Table 1.
Ways of transmission of the hepatitis B virus [14].

HBV is not transmitted through contaminated food or water, insects or other vectors [16]. Sexual transmission and injection drug use account for most transmissions of the virus in low-prevalence regions [17].

Vertical or perinatal transmission of HBV is more common in Asian countries and Oceania regions [14]. Mothers with a high viral load who are not on antiviral treatment are more likely to transmit the virus to their newborn [18]. Infection during childbirth occurs in up to 20% of children born to HBsAg-positive and HBeAg-negative women [19]. While most perinatal infections occur in babies born to chronically infected mothers, those with acute HBV infection in the third trimester are also highly likely to transmit the virus [19].

2.1 Perinatal transmission

In areas with high endemicity, especially Southeast Asia, transmission of HBV from carrier mothers to their children during the perinatal period is the most common cause [20]. HBV infections are more frequent when the mother has both positive HBsAg and HBeAg than in the case of those with positive HBsAg and negative HBeAg [20]. There are three modes of transmission of HBV from infected mothers to infants [21]:

- transplacental transmission (*in utero*)
- congenital transmission during birth
- postnatal transmission during care or through breast milk [21].

Because transplacental transmission occurs antenatally, hepatitis B vaccine and hepatitis B immune globulin (HBIG) cannot block this pathway [16]. Considerable risk of hepatitis B infection in the perinatal period from mothers with acute HBV infection is possible, especially in the third trimester or in the first 2 months after birth [22]. *In utero* transmission is uncommon because HBV does not cross the intact placenta, and the limited number of intrauterine infections is probably due to maternal-fetal blood contact associated with placental abruption [23].

Studies on the transplacental transmission of HBV have suggested two possible mechanisms via the hematogenous route: microrupture of the placenta so that maternal blood infected with high titer HBV enters the fetal circulation and the second mechanism by cell transfer via villous capillary endothelial cells [23]. HBeAg is a serological marker for hepatitis B DNA viral load; thus, hepatitis B virus DNA greater than 200,000 IU/ml in maternal blood determines 100% infection of the fetus [24].

2.2 Sexual transmission

Sexual transmission of hepatitis B is an important source of infection in all areas of the world, but especially in areas of low endemicity (North America), but is increasingly important in areas of high endemicity, as young people adopt a style of "Western" life [25]. Hepatitis B is considered a sexually transmitted disease (STD), and for a long time, gay men were considered to be at the highest risk of infection through sexual contact [26].

However, heterosexual transmission accounts for an increasing proportion of HBV infections [27]. Factors associated with increased risk of HBV infection include unprotected sex, number of sexual partners, and history of other sexually transmitted diseases [26]. Sexual partners of injecting drug users and prostitutes are at particularly high risk of HBV infection [16]. It has been documented in most industrialized countries that HBV infection is found mainly in adolescents and young adults, and sexual transmission is the strongest risk factor for infection, accounting for at least 30 to 50% of acute hepatitis B cases [28]. The risk of chronicity is <5% for sexual transmission [33].

2.3 Parenteral/percutaneous transmission

Parenteral transmission includes injection drug use, blood transfusions and hemodialysis, acupuncture, handling contaminated objects, tattoos, and household contact [29]. In the United States and Western Europe, injection drug use remains a very important mode of transmission of HBV infection (up to 25% of all patients) [16]. The risk of infection increases with the duration of injection drug use [30]. Although the risk of transfusion-associated HBV infection has been greatly reduced since screening blood for HBV, hepatitis C virus (HCV), and HBV vaccination (HIV) markers and excluding donors who engage in high-risk activities, transmission is still possible when donors are in the "serologic window," until the appearance of HBsAg in the blood and only HBV-DNA dosing would make detection possible, but this is an expensive method even for economically developed countries [31].

Obvious sources of infection include HBV-contaminated blood and products, with contaminated surgical instruments being other possible hazards [30]. Parenteral/percutaneous transmission can occur during surgery, after needle stick injuries, intravenous drug use, and after procedures such as body piercing, tattooing, and acupuncture [32].

2.4 Prevention of HBV infection

Reduction of HBV-related chronic liver damage and chronic HBV infection is the primary goal of hepatitis B prevention initiatives [34]. Many effective hepatitis B prevention measures have been partially or fully implemented (**Table 2**) [34]. Three strategies are available to prevent HBV infection: prevention through behavioral changes, passive immunoprophylaxis, and active immunization (vaccination) [35].

2.5 Behavior modification

Sex education, combating drug use, compliance with the rules of asepsis and antisepsis in hospitals and medical units, as well as screening of transfused blood

• included blood donor screening, • plasma-derived product preparation that inactivates the HBV virus, • infection control measures, • the administration of hepatitis B immune globulin after suspected exposure, particularly for infants born to HBsAg-positive women [35].

Table 2.
Prevention of HBV infection [35].

products are methods to combat HBV transmission [16]. Behavior modification is more important in developed countries than in developing countries, where the main route of transmission is vertical (perinatal), for this group, immunoprophylaxis, both passive and active, being more effective [20].

2.6 Passive immunoprophylaxis with HBIG

Hepatitis B immune globulin (HBIG) is a sterile solution of antibodies against hepatitis B [36]. HBIG is prepared from human blood from selected donors who already have a high level of antibodies against hepatitis B and is used in passive immunoprophylaxis [37]. Passive immunoprophylaxis is used in the following situations: newborns of mothers infected with hepatitis B, after accidental injection with objects contaminated with HBV, after sexual exposure, and after liver transplantation [38]. HBIG is an essential component of prophylaxis in HBV-infected patients and liver transplant recipients, which prevents recurrence in up to 80% of cases [39]. Long-term prophylaxis, in high doses of HBIG, has an extremely high cost, so the combined therapy between a nucleoside analog and HBIG is used [39].

2.7 Active immunization (vaccine)

The best way to reduce the prevalence of HBV infection is by vaccination and routine infant vaccination, which has been the main approach in nations in eastern Europe [15]. In 1982, the inactive plasma-derived vaccination, known as the first-generation hepatitis B vaccine, was made accessible [40]. The second-generation HBV recombinant DNA vaccine has been available for general use since 1985 [41]. Both vaccines have been shown to be safe and effective in preventing HBV infection.

In 1991, the World Health Organization (WHO) recommended that vaccination against hepatitis B be included in the national immunization system in countries with hepatitis B carrier prevalence (HBsAg) of 8% or greater by 1995 and in all countries by 1997 [42].

The hepatitis B vaccine has now been available for over 30 years, being a very effective tool for preventing infections among the population [43]. The US implemented universal immunization in 1991 and decreased the incidence of acute infections by 89% in children and adolescents [44]. With the introduction of HBV vaccination on a large scale, the incidence of liver cirrhosis and hepatocellular carcinoma is expected to decrease over the next few decades [45]. Taiwan is one of the early adopters of universal vaccination. Its prevalence of positive surface antigen, that was between 15 and 20%, has reduced to 7% among adolescents and young children [46]. In 2002, 154 countries had routine immunization of infants with the hepatitis B vaccine [47].

Given that anti-HB antibodies can disappear to a substantial extent in those vaccinated, after the initial successful vaccination, a booster dose is required of vaccine, following the administration of the primary course, which is recommended by most national bodies [48]. Results of long-term follow-up studies, along with role assessment of immunological memory among those vaccinated, show that the need to provide booster doses after a successful course is now being questioned in primary immunization [48]. The data collected from the literature show us that long-term protection depends more on immune memory than on the decrease in the titer of antiHBs antibodies [49]. Therefore, to ensure continued access to hepatitis B vaccines worldwide, major efforts are needed to support countries securing sustained funding for immunization programs [49].

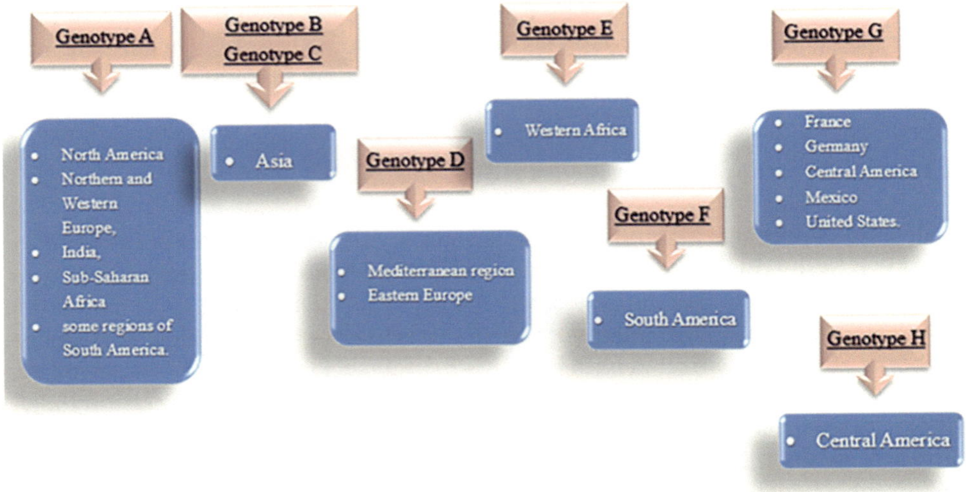

Figure 1.
Hepatitis B genotype and global distribution [29].

3. Hepatitis B genotype

There are eight HBV genotypes grouped from A-H based on the phylogenetic analysis of the complete classification of the viral genome, each with a unique geographic distribution (**Figure 1**) [38]. At the global level, the most widespread types are genotypes A and D. In East Asia, the area with high endemicity, Genotypes B and C are found.

The 8th "H," described last, is found in Central America. Genotype E is found in sub-Saharan Africa, and genotype F is seen in Native Americans [50]. All genotype classes have a common immunodominant region on the HBs antigen which is called "a determinant" [14]. This determinant comprises amino acids 124–147 and is hydrophilic [14]. It is taught to be a form of two major and one minor loop with cysteine disulfide bonds. The "a" determinant primarily targets vaccine-induced neutralizing antibodies, which achieves a common major immunization response to the "a" determinant, with subsequent protection against all HBV subtypes [51].

The response to treatment depends on the genotype, subgroup, and recombination, which can influence the biological characteristics of the virus [38]. A correlation between HBV genotypes and HBeAg clearance, liver damage, and response to IFN treatment has been reported [52]. The prevalence of HBeAg seems higher in patients with genotype C than with genotype B, also, patients with genotype B have lower histological activity scores and genotype C is more prevalence in patients with cirrhosis [52].

4. Coinfection

Due to similar mechanisms of transmission, overlapping patterns of endemicity are seen between HBV and other blood-borne viruses like hepatitis C virus (HCV), hepatitis D virus (HDV), and HIV [29]. Coinfection with these viruses alters the natural course of evolution, and the prognosis is poor compared to HBV monoinfection [53]. Chronic HDV infection is often linked to an ongoing chronic hepatitis, which in approximately 70% of cases develops into cirrhosis within 5–10 years [54]. HBV/HDV coinfection has an estimated three times greater incidence of cirrhosis than those with chronic HBV monoinfection and they have higher risk of early decompensation and the development of hepatocellular carcinoma [38].

Considering the increased risk of complications, prevention of infection in patients with HBV or with HCV or HIV (by HBV vaccination) is of high priority. Of the estimated 240–350 million people living with HBV worldwide, coinfection with HIV is estimated at 0.5–1.5% [55].

In some regions, up to 25% of people are infected with HIV are also infected with HBV. From the point of view of HBV/HCV coinfection, it is estimated that between 7 and 20 million are co-infected, with evidence that this coinfection increases the risk of progression to cirrhosis and HCC [56]. HDV is a satellite RNA virus, which only affects people carrying HBV (5% globally) [57]. Perinatal transmission is less common than for HBV. However, the prevalence of HDV has been shown to be decreasing particularly in South-Eastern Europe, due to improvements in primary prevention of HBV through vaccination, reduction of harm in people who inject drugs and general improvement in socioeconomic conditions [29].

5. Epidemiology of HCC and HBV

Hepatocarcinoma (HCC) is one of the reducible complications of HBV infection, being able to occur in patients with chronic HBV hepatitis, not only in those in the stage of cirrhosis [58]. Compared to uninfected people, the risk of HCC is 100 times higher in those with positive HBsAg and especially in those with high viral replication (much increased HBV-DNA) [59]. The presence of HCC correlates with the geographical prevalence, being higher in Southeast Asia and sub-Saharan Africa (HCC >50 per 100,000 inhabitants) [60]. Genotype also plays a role in the development of HCC, with data from Asia showing that genotype C is associated with more severe liver disease including cirrhosis and HCC, while genotype B is associated with the development of HCC in young and noncirrhotic patients [61].

6. HBV in developing countries

In developing countries, HBV incidence is medium to high, even if the number of chronic HBV carriers has decreased since the introduction of the vaccine in the 1990s [27]. In the sub-Saharan region of Africa, the endemicity of HBV infection exceeds 8% of the general population [62]. There are also countries with <2% endemicity on the African continent, these being Egypt, Algeria and Morocco [63]. In South Africa, the highest rate of hepatitis B infection in children under 10 was 15% [64]. There is evidence to suggest that vertical transmission is more common in Asia than in Africa, related in part to predominant HBV genotypes influencing the likelihood of HBeAg positivity and high levels of HBV-DNA during childbearing years [20]. In China, HBsAg prevalence has decreased from 10 to 1.0% in children under 5 years of age, preventing approximately 16 to 20 million cases of HBV infection through population vaccination [65].

Southeast European nations with intermediate-to-high HBsAg carriage rates include Bulgaria (4%) and Romania (5.6%), as well as Turkey (up to 7%) [66]. On the other hand, the majority of Western and Central Europe, including nations like Belgium, Italy, Germany, the Czech Republic, and Slovakia, have low levels of HBV endemicity (0.5–1%) [67]. The Netherlands, Northern European nations including the UK and Ireland, and Scandinavian nations like Denmark and Finland have the lowest HBV seroprevalence (<0.5) [67].

For Latin America, epidemiological data are insufficient, but according to estimates, almost 12 million people are currently infected with HBV, and the most affected age group is 20–40 years [68]. Nations that cannot yet adopt a universal newborn immunization program must receive support from international organizations to implement this. The WHO Global Hepatitis Strategy, endorsed by all WHO Member States, aims to reduce new hepatitis infections by 90% and deaths by 65% between 2016 and 2030 [69].

Author details

Mariana Mihăilă[1*], Cătălin Ştefan Ghenea[2] and Livia Marieta Negoiță[2]

1 Center of Internal Medicine, Fundeni Clinical Institute, Bucharest, Romania

2 Department of Gastroenterology, Clinical Emergency Hospital of Bucharest, Bucharest, Romania

*Address all correspondence to: m.mihaila@yahoo.com

References

[1] Nayagam S, Thursz M. Strategies for global elimination of chronic HBV infection: 2019 update. Current Hepatology Reports. 2019;**18**(3):300-309. DOI: 10.1007/s11901-019-00478-w

[2] Zhang C, Liu Y, Zhao H, Wang G. Global patterns and trends in total burden of hepatitis B from 1990 to 2019 and predictions to 2030. Clinical Epidemiology. 2022;**14**:1519-1533. DOI: 10.2147/CLEP.S389853

[3] Sagnelli E, Sagnelli C, Pisaturo M, Macera M, Coppola N. Epidemiology of acute and chronic hepatitis B and delta over the last 5 decades in Italy. World Journal of Gastroenterology. 2014;**20**(24):7635-7643. DOI: 10.3748/wjg.v20.i24.7635

[4] Ajuwon BI, Yujuico I, Roper K, Richardson A, Sheel M, Lidbury BA. Hepatitis B virus infection in Nigeria: A systematic review and meta-analysis of data published between 2010 and 2019. BMC Infectious Diseases. 2021;**21**(1):1120. DOI: 10.1186/s12879-021-06800-6

[5] Liang TJ. Hepatitis B: The virus and disease. Hepatology. 2009;**49**(Suppl. 5):13-21. DOI: 10.1002/hep.22881

[6] McGlynn KA, Petrick JL, London WT. Global epidemiology of hepatocellular carcinoma: An emphasis on demographic and regional variability. Clinics in Liver Disease. 2015;**19**(2):223-238. DOI: 10.1016/j.cld.2015.01.001

[7] Rizzo GEM, Cabibbo G, Craxì A. Hepatitis B virus-associated hepatocellular carcinoma. Viruses. 2022;**14**(5):986-1006. DOI: 10.3390/v14050986

[8] Plotkin S, Orenstein W, Offit P, Kathryn ME. Plotkin's Vaccines. 7th ed. Amsterdam: Elsevier; 2018

[9] Schillie S et al. Prevention of hepatitis B virus infection in the United States: Recommendations of the advisory committee on immunization practices. MMWR Recommendations and Reports. 2018;**67**(1):1-31. DOI: 10.15585/mmwr.rr6701a1

[10] Terrault NA, Bzowej NH, Chang K-M, Hwang JP, Jonas MM, Murad MH. AASLD guidelines for treatment of chronic hepatitis B. Hepatology. 2016;**63**(1):261-283. DOI: 10.1002/hep.28156

[11] Kwon SY, Lee CH. Epidemiology and prevention of hepatitis B virus infection. The Korean Journal of Hepatology. 2011;**17**(2):87-95. DOI: 10.3350/kjhep.2011.17.2.87

[12] Genesca J et al. Hepatitis b virus replication in acute hepatitis B, acute hepatitis B virus-hepatitis delta virus coinfection and acute hepatitis delta superinfection. Hepatology. 1987;**7**(3):569-572. DOI: 10.1002/hep.1840070325

[13] Umar M, Hamama-Tul-Bushra SU, Khan HA. HBV perinatal transmission. International Journal of Hepatology. 2013;**2013**:875791. DOI: 10.1155/2013/875791

[14] Katamba C, Philippe CO. Ch. 1. In: Rodrigo L, editor. Epidemiology of Hepatitis B Virus. Rijeka: IntechOpen; 2021

[15] Nelson NP, Easterbrook PJ, McMahon BJ. Epidemiology of hepatitis B virus infection and impact of

vaccination on disease. Clinics in Liver Disease. 2016;**20**(4):607-628. DOI: 10.1016/j.cld.2016.06.006

[16] Hou J, Liu Z, Gu F. Epidemiology and prevention of hepatitis B virus infection. International Journal of Medical Sciences. 2005;**2**(1):50-57. DOI: 10.7150/ijms.2.50

[17] Trickey A et al. The contribution of injection drug use to hepatitis C virus transmission globally, regionally, and at country level: A modelling study. The Lancet Gastroenterology & Hepatology. 2019;**4**(6):435-444. DOI: 10.1016/S2468-1253(19)30085-8

[18] Wong F, Pai R, Van Schalkwyk J, Yoshida EM. Hepatitis B in pregnancy: A concise review of neonatal vertical transmission and antiviral prophylaxis. Annals of Hepatology. 2014;**13**(2):187-195. DOI: 10.1016/s1665-2681(19)30881-6

[19] Duri K et al. Antenatal hepatitis B virus sero-prevalence, risk factors, pregnancy outcomes and vertical transmission rate within 24 months after birth in a high HIV prevalence setting. BMC Infectious Diseases. 2023;**23**(1):736. DOI: 10.1186/s12879-023-08523-2

[20] di Filippo Villa D, Navas M-C. Vertical transmission of hepatitis B virus-an update. Microorganisms. 2023;**11**(5):1140-1160. DOI: 10.3390/microorganisms11051140

[21] Navabakhsh B, Mehrabi N, Estakhri A, Mohamadnejad M, Poustchi H. Hepatitis B virus infection during pregnancy: Transmission and prevention. Middle East Journal of Digestive Diseases. 2011;**3**(2):92-102

[22] Borgia G, Carleo MA, Gaeta GB, Gentile I. Hepatitis B in pregnancy. World Journal of Gastroenterology. 2012;**18**(34):4677-4683. DOI: 10.3748/wjg.v18.i34.4677

[23] Zhao X, Bai X, Xi Y. Intrauterine infection and mother-to-child transmission of hepatitis B virus: Route and molecular mechanism. Infection and Drug Resistance. 2022;**15**:1743-1751. DOI: 10.2147/IDR.S359113

[24] Boucheron P et al. Accuracy of HBeAg to identify pregnant women at risk of transmitting hepatitis B virus to their neonates: A systematic review and meta-analysis. The Lancet Infectious Diseases. 2021;**21**(1):85-96. DOI: 10.1016/S1473-3099(20)30593-4

[25] Atkins M, Nolan M. Sexual transmission of hepatitis B. Current Opinion in Infectious Diseases. 2005;**18**(1):67-72. DOI: 10.1097/00001432-200502000-00011

[26] Meheus A. Teenagers' lifestyle and the risk of exposure to hepatitis B virus. Vaccine. 2000;**18**(Suppl. 1):484-497. DOI: 10.1016/S0264-410X(99)00458-2

[27] Zhang L et al. Status of HBsAg seroprevalence in 15 million rural couples in China: A cross-sectional study. Scientific Reports. 2017;**7**(1):42822. DOI: 10.1038/srep42822

[28] Inoue T, Tanaka Y. Hepatitis B virus and its sexually transmitted infection - an update. Microbial Cell (Graz, Austria). 2016;**3**(9):420-437. DOI: 10.15698/mic2016.09.527

[29] MacLachlan JH, Cowie BC. Hepatitis B virus epidemiology. Cold Spring Harbor Perspectives in Medicine. 2015;**5**(5):a021410. DOI: 10.1101/cshperspect.a021410

[30] Marks LR, Nolan NS, Liang SY, Durkin MJ, Weimer MB. Infectious

complications of injection drug use. The Medical Clinics of North America. 2022;**106**(1):187-200. DOI: 10.1016/j.mcna.2021.08.006

[31] Niederhauser C. Reducing the risk of hepatitis B virus transfusion-transmitted infection. Journal of Blood Medicine. 2011;**2**:91-102. DOI: 10.2147/JBM.S12899

[32] Aljarbou AN. The emergent concern of hepatitis B globally with special attention to Kingdom of Saudi Arabia. International Journal of Health Sciences (Qassim). 2013;**7**(3):333-340. DOI: 10.12816/0006062

[33] Hyams KC. Risks of chronicity following acute hepatitis B virus infection: A review. Clinical Infectious Diseases. 1995;**20**(4):992-100. DOI: 10.1093/clinids/20.4.992

[34] Alter MJ. Epidemiology and prevention of hepatitis B. Seminars in Liver Disease. 2003;**23**(1):39-46. DOI: 10.1055/s-2003-37583

[35] Chang M-H, Chen D-S. Prevention of hepatitis B. Cold Spring Harbor Perspectives in Medicine. 2015;**5**(3):a021493. DOI: 10.1101/cshperspect.a021493

[36] Habib S, Shaikh OS. Hepatitis B immune globulin. Drugs Today (Barc). 2007;**43**(6):379-394. DOI: 10.1358/dot.2007.43.6.1050792

[37] Eke AC, Eleje GU, Eke UA, Xia Y, Liu J. Hepatitis B immunoglobulin during pregnancy for prevention of mother-to-child transmission of hepatitis B virus. Cochrane Database of Systematic Reviews. 2017;**2**(2):CD008545. DOI: 10.1002/14651858.CD008545.pub2

[38] Mihăilă M, Pascu CM, Andrunache A, Ștefan Ghenea C. Ch. 4. In: Parikesit AA, editor. HBV and HCV Infection Prophylaxis in Liver Transplant Recipients. Rijeka: IntechOpen; 2023

[39] Lai Q, Mennini G, Giovanardi F, Rossi M, Giannini EG. Immunoglobulin, nucleos(t)ide analogues and hepatitis B virus recurrence after liver transplant: A meta-analysis. European Journal of Clinical Investigation. 2021;**51**(8):e13575. DOI: 10.1111/eci.13575

[40] Romano L, Zanetti AR. Hepatitis B vaccination: A historical overview with a focus on the Italian achievements. Viruses. 2022;**14**(7):1515-1523. DOI: 10.3390/v14071515

[41] Weinman SA, Taylor R. In: McManus LM, Mitchell RNBTPHD, editors. Viral Hepatitis. San Diego: Academic Press; 2014. pp. 1838-1856

[42] Dassah S et al. Seroconversion of hepatitis B vaccine in young children in the Kassena Nankana district of Ghana: A cross-sectional study. PLoS One. 2015;**10**(12):e0145209. DOI: 10.1371/journal.pone.0145209

[43] Pattyn J, Hendrickx G, Vorsters A, Van Damme P. Hepatitis B vaccines. The Journal of Infectious Diseases. 2021;**224**(12 Suppl 2):S343-S351. DOI: 10.1093/infdis/jiaa668

[44] Chen D-S. Hepatitis B vaccination: The key towards elimination and eradication of hepatitis B. Journal of Hepatology. 2009;**50**(4):805-816. DOI: 10.1016/j.jhep.2009.01.002

[45] Flores JE, Thompson AJ, Ryan M, Howell J. The global impact of hepatitis B vaccination on hepatocellular carcinoma. Vaccine. 2022;**10**(5):793-803. DOI: 10.3390/vaccines10050793

[46] Ni YH et al. Hepatitis B virus infection in children and adolescents in a hyperendemic area: 15 years after

mass hepatitis B vaccination. Annals of Internal Medicine. 2001;**135**(9):796-800. DOI: 10.7326/0003-4819-135-9-200111060-00009

[47] Namgyal P. Impact of hepatitis B immunization, Europe and worldwide. Journal of Hepatology. 2003;**39**(Suppl):1. DOI: 10.1016/s0168-8278(03)00269-1

[48] Bruce MG et al. Antibody levels and protection after hepatitis B vaccine: Results of a 30-year follow-up study and response to a booster dose. The Journal of Infectious Diseases. 2016;**214**(1):16-22. DOI: 10.1093/infdis/jiv748

[49] Puvacić S, Ravlija J, Puvacić Z, Curić I. Long term protection after hepatitis B vaccination. Bosnian Journal of Basic Medical Sciences. 2005;**5**(3):50-53

[50] Sunbul M. Hepatitis B virus genotypes: Global distribution and clinical importance. World Journal of Gastroenterology. 2014;**20**(18):5427-5434. DOI: 10.3748/wjg.v20.i18.5427

[51] Hehle V et al. Potent human broadly neutralizing antibodies to hepatitis B virus from natural controllers. The Journal of Experimental Medicine. 2020;**217**(10):217-227. DOI: 10.1084/jem.20200840

[52] Seo Y, Yano Y. Short- and long-term outcome of interferon therapy for chronic hepatitis B infection. World Journal of Gastroenterology. 2014;**20**(37):13284-13292. DOI: 10.3748/wjg.v20.i37.13284

[53] Singh KP, Crane M, Audsley J, Avihingsanon A, Sasadeusz J, Lewin SR. HIV-hepatitis B virus coinfection: Epidemiology, pathogenesis, and treatment. AIDS. 2017;**31**(15):2035-2052. DOI: 10.1097/QAD.0000000000001574

[54] Da BL, Heller T, Koh C. Hepatitis D infection: From initial discovery to current investigational therapies. Gastroenterology Report. 2019;**7**(4):231-245. DOI: 10.1093/gastro/goz023

[55] Platt L et al. Prevalence and burden of HBV co-infection among people living with HIV: A global systematic review and meta-analysis. Journal of Viral Hepatitis. 2020;**27**(3):294-315. DOI: 10.1111/jvh.13217

[56] Mavilia MG, Wu GY. HBV-HCV coinfection: Viral interactions, management, and viral reactivation. Journal of Clinical and Translational Hepatology. 2018;**6**(3):296-305. DOI: 10.14218/JCTH.2018.00016

[57] Stockdale AJ et al. The global prevalence of hepatitis D virus infection: Systematic review and meta-analysis. Journal of Hepatology. 2020;**73**(3):523-532. DOI: 10.1016/j.jhep.2020.04.008

[58] Ghenea CS, Ștefania Dumitrescu L, Negoita M, Mihaila LA, Constantinescu G. Real-world single-center clinical data on sorafenib in patients with unresectable hepatocellular carcinoma. Journal of Medical Imaging and Radiation Oncology. 2022;**II**:18-26. DOI: 10.53011/JMRO.2022.01.03

[59] Arbuthnot P, Kew M. Hepatitis B virus and hepatocellular carcinoma. International Journal of Experimental Pathology. 2001;**82**(2):77-100. DOI: 10.1111/j.1365-2613.2001.iep0082-0077-x

[60] Chidambaranathan-Reghupaty S, Fisher PB, Sarkar D. Hepatocellular carcinoma (HCC): Epidemiology, etiology and molecular classification. Advances in Cancer Research. 2021;**149**:1-61. DOI: 10.1016/bs.acr.2020.10.001

[61] Zhang Q, Cao G. Genotypes, mutations, and viral load of hepatitis B virus and the risk of hepatocellular carcinoma: HBV properties and hepatocarcinogenesis. Hepatitis Monthly. 2011;**11**(2):86-91

[62] Stockdale AJ et al. Prevalence of hepatitis D virus infection in sub-Saharan Africa: A systematic review and meta-analysis. The Lancet Global Health. 2017;**5**(10):992-1003. DOI: 10.1016/S2214-109X(17)30298-X

[63] Zampino R et al. Hepatitis B virus burden in developing countries. World Journal of Gastroenterology. 2015;**21**(42):11941-11953. DOI: 10.3748/wjg.v21.i42.11941

[64] Moonsamy S, Pillay P, Prabdial-Sing N. Hepatitis B infection status among south Africans attending public health facilities over a five-year period: 2015 to 2019. PLOS Global Public Health. 2023;**3**(9):e0000992. DOI: 10.1371/journal.pgph.0000992

[65] Liang X et al. Reprint of: Epidemiological serosurvey of hepatitis B in China—declining HBV prevalence due to hepatitis B vaccination. Vaccine. 2013;**31**:J21-J28. DOI: 10.1016/j.vaccine.2013.08.012

[66] Ahmad AA et al. Estimating the scale of chronic hepatitis B virus infection among migrants in EU/EEA countries. BMC Infectious Diseases. 2018;**18**(1):34. DOI: 10.1186/s12879-017-2921-8

[67] Hahné SJM, Veldhuijzen IK, Wiessing L, Lim T-A, Salminen M, van de Laar M. Infection with hepatitis B and C virus in Europe: A systematic review of prevalence and cost-effectiveness of screening. BMC Infectious Diseases. 2013;**13**:181. DOI: 10.1186/1471-2334-13-181

[68] Roman S et al. Hepatitis B virus infection in Latin America: A genomic medicine approach. World Journal of Gastroenterology. 2014;**20**(23):7181-7196. DOI: 10.3748/wjg.v20.i23.7181

[69] Cox AL et al. Progress towards elimination goals for viral hepatitis. Nature Reviews. Gastroenterology & Hepatology. 2020;**17**(9):533-542. DOI: 10.1038/s41575-020-0332-6

Chapter 2

HBsAg Prevalence among Conditionally Healthy Population of Russia in 1982–2023: An Attempt at a Systematic Review and Forecasting the Trend

Victor Manuylov and Sergey Netesov

Abstract

Data on the dynamics of HBsAg carriers as well as acute and chronic hepatitis B cases in Russia over the past 30 years were collected. An analysis of the quality of these data is presented, revealing methodology issues in recruiting and screening volunteers. Possible mistakes in analyzing these data are discussed. Analysis of published data in 58 groups of conditionally healthy individuals in Russia showed a rapid decrease in HBsAg prevalence, following the dynamics of hepatitis B incidence. In the 1990s, HBsAg prevalence ranged from 2 to 5% to 10–17% (in different regions), and by 2020, this parameter had decreased to levels from 0.2–0.8% to 2–4%. The incidence of acute hepatitis B during this period decreased from 42 to 0.3 new cases per 100 k/year, while chronic hepatitis B cases decreased from 100 to 20 per 100 k/year. Further measures to propose hepatitis B virus (HBV) eradication are discussed, along with current problems related to declining vaccination.

Keywords: viral hepatitis, hepatitis B virus, prevalence, chronic HBV carriers, HBsAg, Russian federation

1. Introduction

The incidence of hepatitis B in Russia has decreased significantly over the past 20 years [1, 2]. Following a rapid rise in the 1990s, apparently caused by the widespread use of intravenous drugs [3, 4], since the starting of a universal vaccination program against hepatitis B in 2001 [5], the incidence is continuously decreasing (**Figure 1A**). This suggests that the measures taken to prevent the spread of the hepatitis B virus (HBV) have been effective in reducing the number of new cases. In addition to immunization, these efforts included the increased control on intravenous drug import and usage and the extensive implementation and improvement of PCR and ELISA diagnostics for the analysis of donor blood as well as for identifying spontaneously infected individuals.

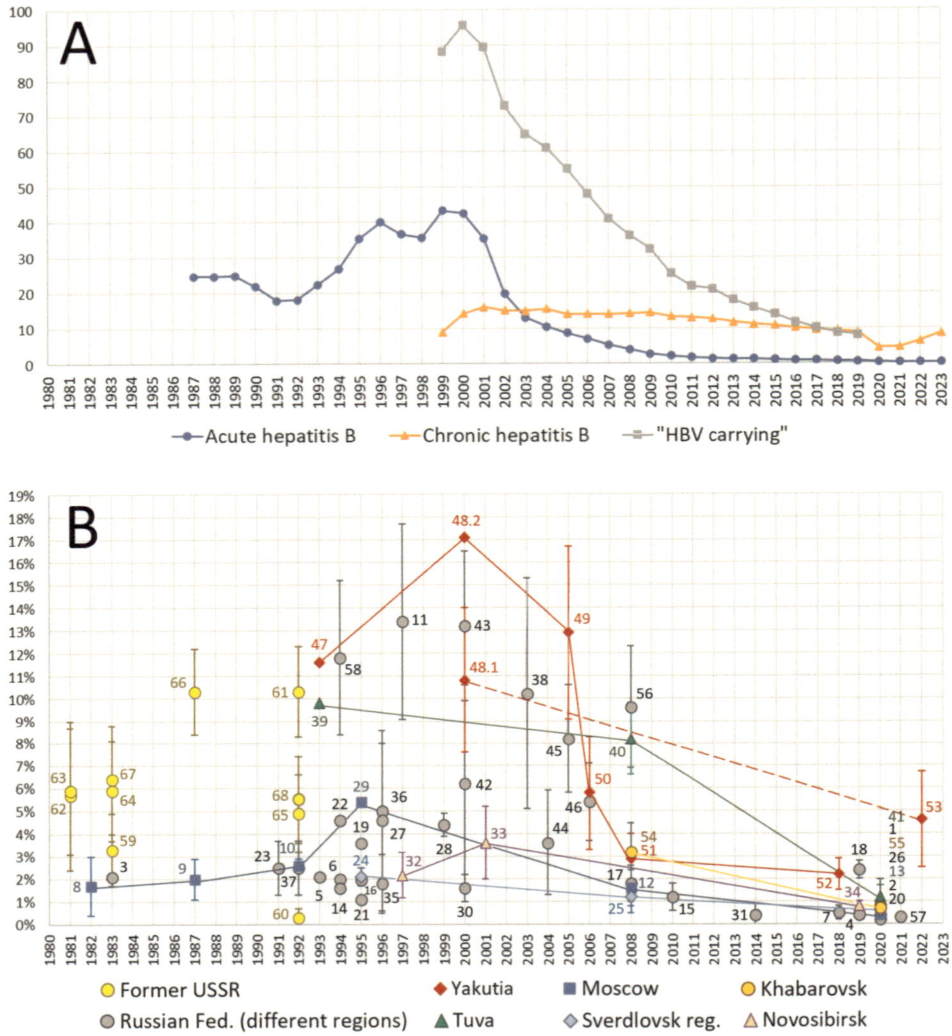

Figure 1.
A: Incidence of hepatitis B in the Russian Federation (1987–2023). The acute hepatitis B (AHB) incidence is depicted by the blue line, chronic hepatitis B (CHB) - by the orange line, and "HBV carrying" by the gray line (until 2019, see the commentaries in the Results section). Data are provided according to [1, 2]. B: The proportion (%) of individuals seropositive for HBsAg in the "conditionally healthy" population of various groups in the Russian Federation (gray points) and other republics of the former USSR (yellow points) over different years. Separately highlighted are Yakutia (red line; the dotted red line connects points in the Arctic zone), Tyva (green line), Moscow and Moscow region (blue), Sverdlovsk region (blue), Novosibirsk region (purple), and Khabarovsk region (orange). The numbers next to the points correspond to the row numbers in ***Table 1****.*

An important question is to what extent the incidence dynamics (i.e., officially registered new cases of hepatitis B) reflect changes in the number of people who are already chronically infected with HBV. From general considerations, the number of chronic HBV carriers should increase quickly following the rise in newly infected individuals (when the incidence is rising), but then decrease much more slowly after the main peak of incidence has passed. This suggestion is based on the facts that the chronic hepatitis B disease is lifelong and, in most cases, cannot be cured but can only be temporarily suppressed with medication. It is often asymptomatic, so the carriers may not know about their illness for some time but can transmit the infection to others. Therefore, the most probable cause of the decrease in the stratum of chronically infected people seems to be their natural death. At the same time, this group of chronic, non-manifest carriers is probably the main reservoir of HBV that infects new individuals, as acute patients release infectious doses of the virus for only a short time. Thus, the rate of decreasing the proportion of chronically HBV-infected people (who are "hidden" in the conditionally healthy population) determines how quickly we can expect the elimination of the pathogen.

The proportion of chronic HBV carriers (the prevalence) at a particular moment cannot be determined solely by analyzing hepatitis B incidence. To assess the prevalence, targeted screenings in groups of a conditionally healthy population are necessary, as asymptomatic chronic HBV carriers who do not know about their infection behave like healthy persons from a clinical and social perspective (although he or she is capable of transmitting the virus accidentally). Fortunately, such local screenings have been performed in the Russian Federation since the early 1980s, when HBV serological diagnosis methods began to be actively introduced into the clinical and epidemiological practice of the Soviet Union. These screening studies experienced a renaissance in the late 1990s with the evolution of molecular tools for detecting and sequencing HBV DNA, and again in the late 2010s when the need for repeated monitoring was realized by several groups of authors simultaneously (**Table 1**). Mostly, such screenings were performed on a regional basis: the proportion of HBV carriers was assessed in groups of a "conditionally healthy" population of particular regions or cities (based on the prevalence of HBsAg, see below). As the data accumulated, it became possible to evaluate the dynamics of the HBV prevalence, i.e., to determine how the number of chronic HBV carriers changes and whether it follows up the curve of hepatitis B incidence. This was the main goal of the present study.

Besides this, we consider it a distinct and important task to publish a comprehensive set of findings on historical HBsAg prevalence in the Russian Federation through an international open-access edition. Many of these findings were previously available only in traditional Russian-language print journals or in even less accessible sources, such as PhD theses or conference reports. This publication makes these data accessible to a broader range of researchers worldwide.

2. Limitations of the study

The works covered by this study were quite diverse (**Table 1**) but often contained typical methodological simplifications that should be discussed prior to the analysis:

1. Most studies only determined HBsAg seroprevalence without confirming positive cases by PCR. While HBsAg is the main diagnostic marker of HBV infection according to both international [34] and Russian [35] recommendations, it is known that the high sensitivity of commercial ELISA kits (which is necessary in their traditional field of use for screening blood donor samples), as well as other factors such as cross-contamination of samples, can sometimes lead to false-positive results. This ultimately results in an overestimation of the proportion of seropositive individuals compared to those in whom HBV DNA is detected [20, 31, 36].

2. In most cases, volunteers were invited as study participants instead of individuals randomly selected from the population who could represent various

#	Region/group	Year(s)	N	HBsAg (+), % [CI 95%]	Additional data about HBV markers (if any available)	Citation
1	Nine regions of Russia, mean	2018–2021	36,145	**0.8%** [0.7–0.9%]	anti-HBc(+):14.2% [13.8–14.6%]; anti-HBs(+)/anti-HBc(−): 39.4% [38.9–39.9%]; anti-HBs(−)/anti-HBc(−): 46.5% [46.0–47.0%]	[6]
2	Kaliningrad	2018–2021	1050	**0.4%** [0.0–0.8%]	anti-HBc(+):17.1% [14.8–19.4%]; anti-HBs(+)/anti-HBc(−): 27.0% [24.3–29.7%]; anti-HBs(−)/anti-HBc(−): 57.5% [54.5–60.5%]	[6]
3	Leningrad	first half of 1980's	NA	**2.1%** (3.4% among children)		[7]
4	St. Petersburg and Leningrad Region	2018–2020	5325	**0.4%** [0.2–0.6%]	anti-HBc(+):10.2% [9.4–11.1%]; anti-HBs(+)/anti-HBc(−): 40.4% [39.1–41.7%]; anti-HBs(−)/anti-HBc(−): 49.4% [48.1–50.7%]	[6]
5	Northwestern and Central Russia, adults	early 1990's	NA	**1.8–2.4%**		[8]
6	Novgorod, blood donors	1990's	NA	**2%**		[3]
7	Belgorod region	2017–2018	1754	**0.5%** [0.2–0.8%]	anti-HBc(+): 17.1% [15.3–18.9%]; anti-HBs(+)/anti-HBc(−): 6.3% [5.2–7.4%]; anti-HBs(−)/anti-HBc(−): 54.4% [52.1–56.7%]	[9]
8	Moscow	1981 (adults), 1982 (children)	100 (adults), 256 (children)	**3.0%** [0–6.3%] (adults) **1.2%** [0–2.5%] (children)	anti-HBs(+): 28.0% [19.2–36.8%] (adults), 2.3% [0.5–4.1%] (children)	[10]

#	Region/group	Year(s)	N	HBsAg (+), % [CI 95%]	Additional data about HBV markers (if any available)	Citation
9	Moscow	1986–1988	1040	**2.0%** [1.1–2.9%], 1.8% among blood donors	anti-HBs(+): 10.0% [8.2–11.8%]; anti-HBc in the absence of HBsAg and anti-HBs: 4.5% [3.2–5.8%]	[11]
10	Moscow, reserve blood donors	before 1992	3000	**2.63%** [2.0–3.2%]	anti-HBs(+): 27.3% [25.7–28.9%]; anti-HBc(+): 28.6% [27.0–30.2%]	[12]
11	Moscow region, young people (16–20 years)	1990–e	NA	**5.4%**		[13]
12	Moscow	2008	1070	**1.6%** [0.8–2.4%]	anti-HBc(+): 13.6% [11.5–15.7%]	[14]
13	Moscow and Moscow region	2018–2021	8480	**0.4%** [0.3–0.5%]	anti-HBc(+): 11.3% [10.6–12.0%]; anti-HBs(+)/anti-HBc(−): 37.5% [36.5–38.5%]; anti-HBs(−)/anti-HBc(−): 51.1% [50.0–52.2%]	[6]
14	Cherepovets (Vologda region), blood donors	1990's	NA	**1.6%**		[3]
15	Arkhangelsk, adults (18–39 years)	2010–2011	1243	**1.2%** [0.6–1.8%]	Among HBsAg-negatives: anti-HBc&anti-HBs(+): 6.7% [5.3–8.1%]; anti-HBs(+)/anti-HBc(−): 46.9% [44.1–49.7%]; anti-HBs(−)/anti-HBc(+): 3.0% [2.1–3.9%]	[15]
16	Vladimir	1990's	947 (208 children up to 6 years, 201–7–14 years, 538 abults)	From **0.9%** (3–6 years) to **3.0%** (40–49 years)		[16]
17	Rostov-on-Don	2008	1001	**1.8%** [1.0–2.6%]	anti-HBc(+): 18.9% [16.5–21.3%]	[14]
18	Dagestan	2018–2020	4853	**2.4%** [2.0–2.8%]	anti-HBc(+): 23.1% [21.9–24.3%]; anti-HBs(+)/anti-HBc(−): 29.8% [28.5–31.1%]; anti-HBs(−)/anti-HBc(−): 47.1% [45.7–48.5%]	[6]

#	Region/group	Year(s)	N	HBsAg (+), % [CI 95%]	Additional data about HBV markers (if any available)	Citation
19	Nalchik, blood donors	1990's	NA	**3.6%**		[3]
20	Tatarstan	2018–2021	823	**0.2%** [0.0–0.5%]	anti-HBc(+): 11.5% [9.3–13.7%]; anti-HBs(+)/anti-HBc(−): 37.1% [33.8–40.4%]; anti-HBs(−)/anti-HBc(−): 51.0% [47.6–54.4%]	[6]
21	Perm, blood donors	1990's	NA	**1.1%**		[3]
22	Komi-Permyak Autonomous Region, доноры	1990's	NA	**4.6%**		[3]
23	Nizhniy Tagil (Sverdlovsk reg.), Bratsk (Irkutsk reg.), reserve blood donors	before 1992	600	**2.5%** [1.3–3.7%]	anti-HBs(+): 28.5% [24.9–32.1%]; anti-HBc(+): 31.7% [27.9–35.4%]	[12]
24	Verkhnyaya Pyshma (Sverdlovsk reg.), adolescents	1990's	2014 (12–14 years), 2263 (15–17 years), 220 (18–20 years)	**1.9%** [1.3–2.5%] (12–14 years) **2.2%** [1.6–2.8%] (15–17 years) **3.6%** [1.1–6.1%] (18–20)	anti-HBs(+): 12.2% [10.8–13.6%] (12–14 years); 20.9% [19.2–22.6%] (15–17 years); 30.4% [24.3–36.5%]	[17]
25	Sverdlovsk region	2008	1029	**1.2%** [0.5–1.9%]	anti-HBc(+): 17.5% [15.2–19.8%]	[14]
26	Sverdlovsk region	2018–2021	935	**0.6%** [0.1–1.1%]	anti-HBc(+): 16.5% [14.2–19.0%]; anti-HBs(+)/anti-HBc(−): 27.7% [24.9–30.7%]; anti-HBs(−)/anti-HBc(−): 55.9% [52.7–59.1%]	[6]
27	Surgut (Khanty-Mansi Autonomous Region)	1995–1996	396 (279 pregnant women and 117 primary blood donors)	**1.8%** [0.5–3.1%]	anti-HBs(+): 21.7% [17.7–25.8%]	[18]

#	Region/group	Year(s)	N	HBsAg (+), % [CI 95%]	Additional data about HBV markers (if any available)	Citation
28	Aboriginals of Siberia, mean value	1992–2006	5657	**4.4%** [3.9–4.9%]		[19]
29	Khanty and Mansi (aboriginal population of Khanty-Mansi Autonomous Region)	1995–1996	108	**4.6%** [0.6–8.6%]	anti-HBs(+): 36.4% [24.8–48.0%] (n = 66)	[18]
30	Yamalo-Nenetsky Autonomous Region, aboriginals (Khants, Komi, Nenets, Selkups)	1992–2006	1647	From **0%** to **1.6%** [1.0–2.2%]		[20–22]
31	Tazovsky district (Yamalo-Nenetsky Autonomous Region)	2013, 2014, 2016	702 (442 children, 162 adults, 98 old age)	**0.4%** [0–0.9%]	anti-HBc(+): 3–7% depending on age	[23]
32	Novosibirsk	1994–1995	1073	**2.2%** [1.3–3.1%]	Additionally HBsAg presence was determined among blood donors, n = 4553/1.1% HBsAg(+)	[24]
33	Novosibirsk	2000–2002	500	**3.6%** [2.0–5.2%]		[25]
34	Novosibirsk region	2018–2020	8323	**0.8%** [0.6–1.0%]	anti-HBc(+): 11.8% [11.1–12.5%]; anti-HBs(+)/anti-HBc(−): 46.7% [45.6–47.8%]; anti-HBs(−)/anti-HBc(−): 41.5% [40.4–42.6%]	[6]
35	Altai Republic (Altaians)	1997	237	**13.4%** [9.1–17.7%]		[26]
36	Altai Republic (Kazakhs)	1992–2000	200	**5.0%** [2.0–8.0%]		[26, 27]
37	Kemerovo	1991–1993	683	**2.5%** [1.3–3.7%]	anti-HBc(+) among HBsAg(−): 20.1% [17.1–23.1%]	[28]
38	Belovsky district (Kemerovo region), Teleuts	2003	137	**10.2%** [5.1–15.3%]		[19]
39	Tyva	early 1990's	NA	**9.8%**		[8]
40	Tyva	2008	1154	**8.2%** [6.6–9.8%]	anti-HBc(+): 46.2% [43.3–49.1%]	[14]

#	Region/group	Year(s)	N	HBsAg (+), % [CI 95%]	Additional data about HBV markers (if any available)	Citation
41	Tyva	2018–2021	1119	**1.2%** [0.6–1.8%]	anti-HBc(+): 31.7% [29.1–34.5%]; anti-HBs(+)/anti-HBc(−): 22.0% [19.6–24.5%]; anti-HBs(−)/anti-HBc(−): 46.0% [43.1–49.0%]	[6]
42	Turukhansky district (Krasnoyarsk reg.), Kets	2000	113	**6.2%** [1.8–10.6%]		[19]
43	Taimyr peninsula, Dolgans, Nganasans	2000	408	**13.2%** [9.9–16.5%]		[19]
44	Irkutsk region, Russians	2003–2005	250	**3.6%** [1.3–5.9%]		[19]
45	Alarsky district (Irkutsk reg.), Buryats	2005	487	**8.2%** [5.8–10.6%]		[19]
46	Nukutsky district (Irkutsk reg.), Buryats	2006	654	**5.4%** [3.7–7.1%]		[19]
47	Yakutia	early 1990's	NA	**11.6%**		[8]
48	Yakutia, different climatic areas	1999–2002	around 5000	**10.8–17.1%** (Arctic zone) – **10.4–23.8%** (rural zone)	The prevalence on anti-HBc was determined for a subgroup (n = 51) of blood donors in Yakutsk (52.9%), and pregnant women (n = 32) in Yakutsk (56.2%)	[29]
49	Yakutia, Evenks (aboriginals)	2005–2006	301	**12.9%** [9.1–16.7%]	anti-HBs(+): 51.1% [45.5–56.7%] anti-HBc(+): 76% [71.2–80.8%]	[30]
50	Yakutia, Neryungri city (non-aboriginals)	2005–2006	329	**5.8%** [3.3–8.3%]	anti-HBs(+): 23.5% [18.9–28.1%] anti-HBc(+): 14.6% [10.8–18.4%]	[30]
51	Yakutia	2008	968	**2.9%** [1.8–4.0%]	anti-HBc(+): 42.5% [39.4–45.6%]	[14]
52	Yakutia	2017–2018	1072	**2.2%** [1.3–3.1%]	anti-HBc(+): 29.4% [26.7–32.2%]; anti-HBs(+)/anti-HBc(−): 38.4% [35.6–41.4%]; anti-HBs(−)/anti-HBc(−): 69.4% [66.6–72.1%]	[9]

#	Region/group	Year(s)	N	HBsAg (+), % [CI 95%]	Additional data about HBV markers (if any available)	Citation
53	Yakutia (Momsky discrict, Arctic zone)	2022	367	**4.6%** [2.5–6.7%]	anti-HBc(+): 59.4% [54.4–64.4%]	[31]
54	Khabarovsk region	2008	995	**3.2%** [2.1–4.3%]	anti-HBc(+): 21.0% [18.5–23.5%]	[14]
55	Khabarovsk region	2018–2021	5237	**0.7%** [0.5–0.9%]	anti-HBc(+): 14.1% [13.2–15.0%]; anti-HBs(+)/anti-HBc(−): 47.3% [45.9–48.7%]; anti-HBs(−)/anti-HBc(−): 38.7% [37.4–40.0%]	[6]
56	Chukotka	2008	463	**9.6%** [6.9–12.3%] (11.6% among aboriginals and **1.3%** among non-aboriginals)		[32]
57	Chukotka, pregnant women	2020–2022	4495	**0.3%** (initially HBsAg-positive); **3.1%** (those who has been diagnosed as HBV-infected before)		Report on sanitary survey, data unpublished
58	Kamchatka	1994–1995	348	**11.8%** [8.4–15.2%]	anti-HBs(+): 35.9% [30.9–40.9%]	[33]
				The former USSR republics		
59	Tallin (Estonia)	1983	331 (adults), 152 (children)	**4.8%** [2.5–7.1%] (adults), **0%** (children)	anti-HBs(+): 27.2% [22.4–32.0%] (adults), 5.3% [1.7–8.9%] (children)	[10]
60	Riga (Latvia), Kaunas (Lithuania), reserve blood donors	до 1992	642	**0.3%** [0–0.7%]	anti-HBs(+): 29.7% [26.2–33.2%] anti-HBc(+): 26.1% [22.7–29.5%]	[12]
61	Moldova, reserve blood donors	до 1992	900	**10.3%** [8.3–12.3%]	anti-HBs(+): 53.7% [50.4–57.0%] anti-HBc(+): 62.5% [59.3–65.7%]	[12]
62	Zaporozhye (Ukraine)	1981	100 (adults), 93 (children)	**5.0%** [0.7–9.3%] (adults), **6.5%** [1.5–11.5%] (children)	anti-HBs(+): 23.0% [14.8–31.2%] (adults), 14.0% [6.9–21.1%] (children)	[10]

#	Region/group	Year(s)	N	HBsAg (+), % [CI 95%]	Additional data about HBV markers (if any available)	Citation
63	Tbilisi (Georgia)	1981 (adults), 1982 (children)	212 (adults), 57 (children)	**6.1%** [2.9–9.3%] (adults), **5.3%** [0–11.1%] (children)	anti-HBs(+): 30.7% [24.5–26.9%] (adults), 15.8% [6.3–25.3%] (children)	[10]
64	Ashgabat (Turkmenistan)	1983	323 (adults), 135 (children)	**5.6%** [3.1–8.1%] (adults), **6.7%** [2.5–10.9%] (дети)	anti-HBs(+): 33.4% [28.3–38.5%] (adults), 19.3% [12.6–26.0%] (children)	[10]
65	Tashkent (Uzbekistan), Bishkek (former Frunze, Kyrgyzstan), reserve blood donors	before 1992	645	**4.9%** [3.2–6.6%]	anti-HBs(+): 27.3% [23.9–30.7%] anti-HBc(+): 39.8% [36.0–43.6%]	[12]
66	Osh (Kyrgyzstan)	1986–1988	979	**10.3%** [8.4–12.2%]	anti-HBs(+): 22.4% [19.8–25.0%]; anti-HBc(+) in the absence of HBsAg and anti-HBs: 14% [11.8–16.2%]	[11]
67	Alma-Ata (Kazakhstan)	1983	311 (adults), 97 (children)	**6.1%** [3.4–8.8%] (adults), **7.2%** [2.1–12.3%] (children)	anti-HBs(+): 37.0% [31.6–42.4%] (adults), 19.3% [18.9–36.7%] (children)	[10]
68	Uralsk (Northwestern Kazakhstan)	1991–1993	579	**5.5%** [3.6–7.4%]	anti-HBc(+) among HBsAg-negative persons: 22.2% [18.7–25.7%]	[28]

Table 1.
Proportions of HBsAg carriers in "conditionally healthy" populations of the Russian Federation and other republics of the former USSR across different years based on published sources (from West to East and from past to present).

social, economic, and behavioral cohorts. This could lead to an underestimation of the determined HBV prevalence in the studied group (e.g., regional). First, inviting volunteers usually does not attract participants from marginal strata of society, who are not numerous but are much more often infected [4]. Second, researchers are often specifically interested in studying HBV carriers who are "hidden" among a "healthy" population. Consequently, they sometimes restrict the participation of individuals who have already been aware of their positive status regarding viral hepatitis and/or other parenteral infections. The presence of such infections in the anamnesis might be set as an exclusion criterion for potential participants, and thus, these individuals are not included in the group statistics. However, we assume that the systematic factors mentioned in this paragraph and the paragraph above affected the data of all studies in the same way and, thus, may not be taken into account in assessing the overall trend.

3. Epidemiological heterogeneity of the study groups and, sometimes, a lack of data complicate joint analysis. Researchers tend to explore groups of volunteers that are easier accessible to them, which cannot always be directly compared to each other (e.g., by age of participants; some authors include children, while others do not). A few sources do not indicate the exact year the samples were collected (an extended period is indicated, see **Table 1**); some of them do not report the size of the study group (only the proportion of HBsAg carriers is indicated, which does not allow to calculate a confidence interval). In extreme cases, there are data available only regarding the HBsAg prevalence in significantly biased cohorts of the "conditionally healthy" population, such as newly recruited or even long-term blood donors or pregnant women (as reflected in **Table 1**). The heterogeneity of the groups studied by different authors is one of the main factors complicating their comparative analysis. Readers should be aware that the data discussed may have been obtained from vastly different populations (with the common feature that they do not include known HBV carriers). Nonetheless, we hope that the inclusion of a significant number of studies and groups in the analysis can help mitigate the influence of random, multidirectional factors on the overall estimate of the dynamics of HBsAg carrier proportions.

3. Methodology

Information for our analysis was collected both by querying the PubMed database (e.g., "HBV Russia," "HBsAg USSR," and derivatives) and by searching in classical libraries for print versions of sources referred to by the authors of articles indexed by PubMed. In total, we obtained information on HBsAg prevalence in 58 regional groups across the Russian Federation over different years, published in 30 sources (**Table 1**). As we also collected additional data that may be of interest to other researchers, such as the prevalence of antibodies to HBV antigens, we included these findings in **Table 1** but do not discuss them in the main text of the article. In addition, several studies published before 1992 included data not only from regions within the modern Russian Federation but also from 10 groups in other republics of the former USSR. We have included this information in **Table 1**, but did not aim to study HBsAg prevalence in these countries in subsequent years.

The data from **Table 1** were used to construct **Figure 1B**, which is a scatter plot showing the HBsAg prevalence in regional groups of the "conditionally healthy" population over different years. For the graph construction (**Figure 1A, B**), Microsoft Excel 2021 was used. If the size of the surveyed group was known, a confidence interval (CI) for the proportion of the qualitative trait was added to the point in **Figure 1B** (95% CI; recalculated using the binomial distribution in all cases). If the exact year of sample collection was unknown, the corresponding point in **Figure 1B** was placed at the border of the interval for one-sided intervals (e.g., "before 1992"); for two-sided intervals, it was placed in the middle (e.g., for the interval "1990s," the point was placed in 1995); for even intervals, the nearest even year to the mean was used as a point. In some cases, the datapoints for time intervals were shifted for a year to the right or left to avoid overlap on the diagram. If repeated data were available for a particular region over several years, the corresponding points in **Figure 1B** were connected with colored lines.

We deliberately did not calculate a resulting curve of "average" values from different regions for the same year. The reasons were as follows: First, as mentioned, not all the groups' sizes were originally known, so we could not account for their contribution to the "average" value. Second, the populations of distinct regions differ significantly in HBV prevalence (and, therefore, in epidemiological characteristics), making it impractical to combine them (for more details, see [6, 37]). Instead, we believe it is more expedient to evaluate the scatter and character of the entire cloud of the points over time.

4. Results

4.1 Hepatitis B incidence dynamics in Russia over the past 35 years

Figure 1A represents the officially registered incidence of hepatitis B in the entire Russian population from 1987 to 2023 [1, 2]. The incidence of acute hepatitis B (AHB) at the beginning of this period remained at the level of 20–25 cases per 100,000 population, then quickly increased to approximately 40 cases per 100,000 by the mid-1990s. By the end of the 1990s, it had reached a historical maximum of 42–43 cases per 100,000. During these same years, statistics began to register cases of chronic hepatitis B (CHB) and, separately, "HBV carrying," which also showed peaks in the late 1990s. (According to the Russian classification, "HBV carrying" means the persistence of HBsAg in the patient's blood for at least 6 months in the absence of symptoms of liver pathology [35]). In particular, the cumulative incidence of CHB and "HBV carrying" reached its highest known value in 2000 at 109.9 cases per 100,000 population. Since 2001, after the universal vaccination program began [5], along with intensified efforts to combat illegal drug use and general economic improvements in the Russian Federation, the incidence naturally began to fall. The most significant decrease was observed until the early 2010s, when the incidence of AHB dropped below the threshold of 2 cases per 100,000. After that, the decreasing in AHB incidence asymptotically slowed, reaching 0.3 cases per 100,000 by 2023 (**Figure 1A**). The decrease in the incidence of CHB and "HBV carrying" was more gradual, and by 2019, their cumulative value was around 20 cases per 100,000 population (in **Figure 1A**, the curves of CHB and "HBV carrying" must be added to each other to obtain the total yearly value). From 2019 onward, data on "HBV carriage" were no longer published, while the incidence of CHB alone was 8.45 cases per 100,000 in 2023 (**Figure 1B**) [38].

At first glance, the decrease in detected cases of "HBV carrying" seems to reflect a proportional reduction in the infectious-active stratum of asymptomatic HBV carriers, which we aimed to study. However, such an assumption does not seem entirely justified to us. Indeed, the new cases of acute hepatitis B are registered every year, so their dynamics truly reflect the activity of the infectious process in the population. In contrast, an HBV carrier is registered once in his or her lifetime and is not included in subsequent years' statistics, and we do not know exactly how long the carrier remains infectious until death. Therefore, data on the registration of new cases alone are insufficient to estimate the total number of infected people or to determine the rate of its decrease. Answers to these questions can only be obtained through population monitoring studies, which involve direct measurements of the proportion of people infected with HBV (or, simplified, the proportion of the HBsAg-positive carriers) in the general population.

4.2 Dynamics of the HBsAg prevalence in Russia

The published results of HBsAg prevalence monitoring in the Russian Federation (as well as in several other former USSR republics in the 1980s; see below) are summarized in **Table 1** and **Figure 1B**. It is even visually evident that the envelope curve representing the proportions of HBsAg-seropositive carriers (outlining the upper values determined in different groups for the same years) surprisingly accurately follows the hepatitis B incidence curve (**Figure 1A**). Indeed, until the early 1990s, the HBsAg prevalence was recorded at a level of 2–3% across the Russian Federation (the gray and blue points in **Figure 1B** before 1992). In several urban communities—such as Novgorod, Cherepovets, Vladimir, Nalchik, Perm, Surgut, and Kemerovo—a low prevalence rate (1–2%) apparently persisted throughout the first half of the 1990s, despite the sharp rise in hepatitis B incidence in the rest of the country (**Table 1**, **Figure 1B**). However, when discussing these low-endemic city groups in the early 1990s, it is important to note that, first, the year of sample collection is not always known, and second, many of the corresponding groups included reserve blood donors (**Table 1**) [3], who are screened repeatedly and therefore generally have a lower prevalence of parenteral infections.

Starting from 1991 or 1992, significantly larger proportions of HBsAg-seropositive individuals began to be identified in many groups—up to 10% or more (**Figure 1B**). This trend reached a maximum around the year 2000, which is the period when the highest incidence rates of all forms of hepatitis B were recorded (**Figure 1A**). To be fair, we cannot state confidently that there were no highly endemic groups in the USSR before the beginning of the 1990s, when the rapid growth in the number of HBV-infected people occurred. The highest known values of HBsAg prevalence were reported in the mid- and late 1990s in relatively isolated national and/or regional groups of Siberia and the Far East, which apparently have their own epidemiological specifics regarding HBV spreading. For example, in the Republic of Sakha (Yakutia) during those years, HBsAg prevalence was recorded at 10.4–23.8% depending on the region; in the Tyva Republic, up to 9.8%; in the Altai Republic and Taimyr Peninsula, more than 13%; in the Chukotka Peninsula, 9.6%, etc. (see **Table 1**). It is likely that during Soviet times, these groups had not yet been studied as thoroughly as they were later, and for this reason, we do not see a "cloud" of high HBsAg prevalence points for them in the 1980s. This assumption is indirectly confirmed by the high rates of HBsAg prevalence determined in the 1980s in other republics of the former USSR, at levels of 5–6% (Ukraine, Georgia, Turkmenistan, Uzbekistan, Kazakhstan) and even 10% (Moldova, Kyrgyzstan; see the lower part of **Table 1** and yellow points in **Figure 1B**).

However, we can definitely state that in almost all regional groups where repeated monitoring was conducted over different years, the prevalence of HBsAg in 2018–2021 has become significantly lower (statistically speaking) than at previous points around 2008 or earlier (in **Figure 1B**, values obtained from different studies for the same region are connected by lines of the same color). This trend was observed not only in national groups, such as the population of the Tuva Republic, where HBsAg prevalence was 8.2 ± 1.6% in 2008 and dropped to 1.2 ± 0.6% in 2020 ($p < 0.001$, **Table 1**), but also in large urban communities with diverse geographical, climatic, and socio-economic conditions. For instance, in Moscow, HBsAg prevalence decreased from 1.6 ± 0.8% in 2008 to 0.4 ± 0.1% in 2020; in Novosibirsk, it fell from 3.6 ± 1.6% in 2001 to 0.8 ± 0.2% in 2020; and in Khabarovsk, it declined from 3.2 ± 1.1% in 2001 to 0.7 ± 0.2% in 2020 (in all these cases, the differences were significant, $p < 0.001$). The exception was the Sverdlovsk region, where the incidence of HBsAg in 2020 (0.6 ± 0.5%) was not statistically different from that in 2008 (1.2 ± 0.7%) but was still significantly lower than the lowest value reported in the 1990s (1.9 ± 0.6%, $p < 0.01$, **Table 1**).

4.3 The republic of Yakutia: From highest to low HBsAg prevalence

The dynamics of HBsAg prevalence in the large Republic of Yakutia (**Figure 1B**, red line) deserves special discussion. In this region, the proportion of HBsAg carriers among the conditionally healthy population in 2018 (2.2 ± 0.6%) did not differ significantly from the previous known value (2008, 2.9 ± 1.1%) but was significantly lower than the reported values for 2005–2006 for both the indigenous population (12.1 ± 3.8%) and the urban (newly arrived) population (5.8 ± 2.5%, **Table 1**). However, the most recent publication [31] reported the HBsAg prevalence in Yakutia in 2022 at 4.6 ± 2.1%, which appears to violate the common trend of decreasing HBsAg carrier proportions in all surveyed groups (**Figure 1A**). At the time, it should be noted that the population of Yakutia is very diverse in terms of HBV prevalence [29, 30]. The mentioned value of 4.6% [31] was obtained in the Momsky region of the Arctic zone in 2022, while lower values—2.2% in 2018 [9] and 2.9% in 2008 [14]—were reported in the more southern regions of the so-called "agriculture zone," including the city of Yakutsk. For previous values of HBsAg prevalence specifically in the Arctic zone, we have data from the neighboring Abyisky district, where in the period of 1999–2002, the HBsAg prevalence was reported at 10.8 ± 3.2% [29]. This was significantly higher than the discussed point of 4.6 ± 2.1% in the same Arctic zone in 2022 [31]. Thus, even in the highly endemic Arctic zone of Yakutia, a significant decrease in the proportion of HBsAg carriers has occurred (see points connected by a red dotted line in **Figure 1B**), in accordance with the general trend throughout the country.

In general, after 2008, no further reports have been published on the rise of the HBsAg prevalence anywhere in Russia (remember, we are discussing the "conditionally healthy" population, not risk groups). By 2018–2021, the average seroprevalence of HBsAg in the country was already estimated at 0.2–0.8% [6], as shown in **Figure 1B**. There are still a few national republics where the HBsAg prevalence has been reported at moderately high levels recently (for example, Dagestan with a rate of 2.4% in 2019–2020, or the previously discussed Yakutia with rates of 2.2–4.6% in 2018–2022, **Table 1**), but even these values are markedly lower than those in the 1990s.

5. Discussion

Thus, the decline in HBsAg prevalence appears to have almost paralleled the decrease in hepatitis B incidence (**Figure 1A, B**). One potential reason for the reduction in the large and seemingly time-stable population of infectious HBV carriers could be their relatively rapid mortality from various causes. Many individuals infected with HBV during the 1990s were drug addicts and had correspondingly elevated risks of mortality from all causes. According to [4], at least 22% of chronically HBV-infected individuals in Siberian cities before 2002 openly admitted injecting drug use (with risk ratios from 2.7 to 27 depending on the subgroup). Since the 2000s, sexual transmission of HBV has become the dominant risk factor (after "unknown causes"), being responsible for 13–30% of all new hepatitis B cases, while drug use remains a likely cause in only about 10% of newly infected patients [39, 40]. Therefore, if the infectious stratum were to increase again, then, due to changes in the behavior of modern HBV carriers, we should not expect a subsequent decrease as rapid as we could observe in the recent past (**Figure 1B**).

Finally, we might face the probable effect described in the "Background" section of this article: the exclusion from late 2010s' studies of people who have already known about their infectious status (or their self-decision not to participate). It is also likely that healthcare in the Russian Federation has reached a level where most HBV carriers are identified quickly after infection. However, this, in our opinion, does not affect the general conclusions. The primary risk of the new HBV invasions comes not from the entire stratum of infected individuals, but specifically from those who are not under specialist supervision, are unaware of their infectious status, and thus take no special measures to prevent virus transmission. The clearly observed reduction in the proportion of these "unconscious" carriers (**Figure 1B**) is an extremely positive trend. If it is possible to reduce the size of this stratum to zero (so every infected person has been aware of his or her status), then we can start to talk about the approaching victory over HBV in Russia—even if the remaining cohort of patients with CHB will persist for many years under the care and control of medical specialists. Of course, it is crucially important to educate all chronically infected individuals with HBV about the necessary restrictions in behavior and habits to prevent further virus transmission.

However, further reduction in HBV prevalence is only possible with increased control over vaccination. By the end of 2021, official data indicated that 109.6 million people in Russia (approximately 75% of the total population of around 146 million) had received a complete course of the hepatitis B vaccine [38]. Despite this, the proportion of people carrying a protective anti-HBsAg IgG's titer (≥10 mIU/ml) in the general population of Russia was, according to various estimates, no more than 66.4–70% depending on the region (study 2017–2019, which included more than 40,000 participants annually [41]) or even as low as 53.6% (2018–2021 study of 36,000 volunteers from 9 regions [6]). This suggests, at least, that not all individuals who receive the vaccine acquire protective immunity (or their immunity is not lifelong), and undervaccinated groups should be identified and boosted.

Additionally, we must not underestimate the impact of anti-vaccination movements, which have led to a noticeable increase in the proportion of unvaccinated newborns in Russia. According to Ref. [42], in 2016–2017, vaccination schedules were violated in 15.7% of children during their first year of life, with 4.9% remaining completely unvaccinated and 10.8% not receiving vaccinations for all the infections listed in the Russian National Vaccination Calendar. Parental prejudice against vaccination accounted for 24.4% of refusals specifically against hepatitis B vaccination [42]. Indirect evidence suggests that the COVID-19 pandemic further fueled anti-vaccination sentiments in Russian society, a situation that urgently requires study and intervention. At a minimum, it is necessary to enhance the postgraduate education of pediatricians and family doctors and to renew efforts in educating parents of new-borns about the importance of vaccination.

6. Conclusion

Until now, we have lacked objective information on how quickly or slowly the size of the infectious stratum of chronic hepatitis B virus carriers is changing in Russia. Our understanding has been based on general assumptions, primarily that chronic hepatitis B is typically a lifelong condition, often asymptomatic and unnoticed by the infected individual. Therefore, the number of HBV carriers may decrease very slowly, mainly through their natural mortality. Considering that many of those infected with hepatitis B during the 1990s—when incidence rates were at their peak—were young people (due to their higher propensity for risky behavior [3, 4]), we could expect this large infectious stratum to persist in society, potentially spreading the virus for many decades. This could have significantly delayed the planned elimination of HBV in Russia.

However, our analysis of long-term publications on HBsAg screening in various regions of Russia revealed that the proportion of HBsAg-positive carriers among the conditionally healthy population, which indeed peaked in the early 2000s, began to rapidly decline almost immediately after the primary wave of morbidity subsided (**Figure 1**). The trends observed in subsequent years clearly demonstrate the infectious stratum's capacity to decrease in response to anti-epidemic measures. This gives us hope that eliminating hepatitis B in the foreseeable future is a realistic goal. Nevertheless, achieving this goal will require the targeted identification and boosting of under immunized groups within the population, which still persist despite mass vaccination efforts.

Acknowledgments and funding

This study was funded by the state assignment for research at Novosibirsk State University, project No. FSUS-2020-0035.

The authors thank Dr. Vladimir Chulanov for providing detailed data on hepatitis B incidence in various regions of Russia.

Conflict of interest

The authors declare no conflict of interest.

Author details

Victor Manuylov* and Sergey Netesov
Novosibirsk State University, Novosibirsk, Russia

*Address all correspondence to: victormanuilov@yandex.ru

References

[1] Federal Service for Supervision of Consumer Rights Protection and Human Welfare. State Report on the State of Sanitary and Epidemiological Well-Being of the Population in the Russian Federation in 2016. Moscow: Federal Service for Supervision of Consumer Rights Protection and Human Welfare; 2017. 220 p. (Russian). Available from: https://www.rospotrebnadzor.ru/upload/iblock/0b3/gosudarstvennyy-doklad-2016.pdf

[2] Federal Service for Supervision of Consumer Rights Protection and Human Welfare. State Report on the State of Sanitary and Epidemiological Well-Being of the Population in the Russian Federation in 2023. Moscow: Federal Service for Supervision of Consumer Rights Protection and Human Welfare; 2024. 364 p. (Russian). Available from: https://rospotrebnadzor.ru/documents/details.php?ELEMENT_ID=27779

[3] Shakhgil'dian IV, Mikhailov MI, Onishchenko GG. Parenteral Viral Hepatitis (Epidemiology, Diagnosis, Prevention). Moscow: State Educational Establishment VUNMC Ministry of Health of the Russian Federation; 2003. 384 p. (Russian)

[4] Kochneva GV. Parenteral viral hepatitis in the Siberian regions of Russia [thesis]. Koltsovo: SSC VB Vector; 2010. (Russian)

[5] Order of the Ministry of Health of the Russian Federation On the national calendar of preventive vaccinations and the calendar of preventive vaccinations for epidemic indications No. 229, dated June 27, 2001 (Russian). Available from: https://normativ.kontur.ru/document?moduleId=1&documentId=122191

[6] Asadi Mobarkhan FA, Manuylov VA, Karlsen AA, Kichatova VS, Potemkin IA, Lopatukhina MA, et al. Post-vaccination and post-infection immunity to the hepatitis B virus and circulation of immune-escape variants in the Russian Federation 20 years after the start of mass vaccination. Vaccine. 2023;**11**:430. DOI: 10.3390/vaccines11020430

[7] Mukomolov SL, Anan'ev VA, Shliakhtenko LI, Nechaev VV, Evdokimova TV. Epidemiological characteristics and the importance of carriers of the surface antigen of the hepatitis B virus (HBsAg). Journal of Microbiology, Epidemiology and Immunobiology. 1984;**12**:76-80. (Russian)

[8] Shakhgil'dian IV, Onishchenko GG, Khukhlovich PA, Anan'ev VA, Kuzin SN, Klimenko SM. Study results and the unresolved problems in the epidemiology and prevention of parenteral viral hepatitis in Russia. Journal of Microbiology, Epidemiology and Immunobiology. 1994;**5**:26-32. (Russian)

[9] Kyuregyan KK, Kichatova VS, Isaeva OV, Potemkin IA, Malinnikova EY, Lopatukhina MA, et al. Coverage with timely administered vaccination against hepatitis B virus and its influence on the prevalence of HBV infection in the regions of different endemicity. Vaccines (Basel). 2021;**9**(2):82. DOI: 10.3390/vaccines9020082

[10] Vyazov SO, Kompaniets AA, Ananyev VA, Listovskaya EK, Dardik FG, Pirozhkova ZP, et al. Detection of HBsAg anti-HBs in healthy population of various cities of the USSR. Voprosy Virusologii. 1985;**2**:231-233. (Russian)

[11] Yashina TL, Favorov MO, Shakhgil'dian IV, Firsova SN, Eraliev AE,

Zhukova LD, et al. The prevalence of the markers of viral hepatitis B and delta among the population in regions differing in the level of morbidity. Voprosy Virusologii. 1992;**4**:194-196. (Russian)

[12] Somova AV, Golosova TV, Margolina AN, Bagryantseva SY. Serodiagnosis of viral hepatitis C and B among various population groups. Voprosy Virusologii. 1992;**4**:191-194. (Russian)

[13] Frolova GS. Optimization of the vaccination scheme against hepatitis B in modern conditions [thesis]. Moscow: Research Center for Children Health of Russian Academy of Medical Sciences; 1999. (Russian)

[14] Klushkina VV, Kyuregyan KK, Kozhanova TV, Popova OE, Dubrovina PG, Isaeva OV, et al. Impact of universal hepatitis B vaccination on prevalence, infection-associated morbidity and mortality, and circulation of immune escape variants in Russia. PLoS One. 2016;**11**(6):e0157161. DOI: 10.1371/journal.pone.0157161

[15] Balaeva T, Grjibovski AM, Samodova O, Sannikov A, Klouman E. Seroprevalence of markers of hepatitis B virus infection, associated factors, and vaccination status in young adults in Arkhangelsk, Northwest Russia: A population-based cross-sectional study. International Journal of Environmental Research and Public Health. 2018;**15**(9): 1905. DOI: 10.3390/ijerph15091905

[16] Kuzin SN, Lisitsina EV, Samokhvalov EI, Shakhgil'dian IV, Kuzina LE, Manina TN, et al. Distribution of hepatitis C and individual genotypes of the hepatitis C virus in a region with moderate activity of the epidemic process. Voprosy Virusologii. 1999;**2**:79-82. (Russian)

[17] Kuznetsova IO. Assessment of the impact of vaccination against hepatitis B in adolescents, newborns and people at risk on the activity of the epidemic process of the hepatitis B virus infection [thesis]. Moscow: D.I. Ivanovsky Research Institute of Virology; 1999. (Russian). Available from: https://viewer.rsl.ru/ru/rsl01000308449?page=1&rotate=0&theme=white

[18] Bakhlykova NY. The prevalence of hepatitis B and C markers among the population and individual risk groups in the middle Ob region [thesis]. Moscow: Central Research Institute of Epidemiology; 1998. (Russian)

[19] Manuylov VA, Osipova LP, Netesova IG, Chub EV, Bezuglova LV, Norder H, et al. The prevalence of HBsAg subtypes and HBV genotypes in native population groups of Siberia. Molecular Genetics, Microbiology and Virology. 2015;**30**:30-38. DOI: 10.3103/S089141681501005X

[20] Manuilov VA, Netesova IG, Osipova LP, Shustov AV, Bayandin RB, Kochneva GV, et al. Genetic variability of hepatitis B virus isolates in the population of the Shuryshkarsky district of the Yamalo-Nenets autonomous Okrug. Molecular Genetics, Microbiology and Virology. 2005;**4**: 30-34. (Russian)

[21] Netesova IG, Swenson PD, Osipova LP, Kalashnikova TV, Netesov SV, Favorov MO. Subtypes of HBsAg of hepatitis B virus in the Western Siberia. Voprosy Virusologii. 2004;**1**:17-20. (Russian)

[22] Dobrodeeva LK, Kornienko EB, Petrenya NN, Lutfalieva GT, Schegoleva LS, Demeneva LV, et al. A unique seroepidemiological pattern of HBV, HCV and HTLV-I in Nenets and Komi in northwestern Russia. Asian

Pacific Journal of Cancer Prevention. 2005;**6**:342-345. Available from: https://journal.waocp.org/?sid=Entrez:PubMed&id=pmid:16235997&key=2005.6.3.342

[23] Bezuglova LV, Osipova LP, Sergeeva EI, Deliy IV, Tabikhanova LE, Netesov SV, et al. Markers of viral hepatitis B in blood plasma samples of the indigenous population of the Russian far north. HBV genotypes and subtypes HBsAg. Molecular Genetics, Microbiology and Virology. 2022;**40**:41-48. DOI: 10.17116/molgen20224003141

[24] Reshetnikov OV, Khryanin AA, Teinina TR, Krivenchuk NA, Zimina IY. Hepatitis B and C seroprevalence in Novosibirsk, western Siberia. Sexually Transmitted Infections. 2001;**77**:463. DOI: 10.1136/sti.77.6.463

[25] Bayandin RB, Shustov AV, Kochneva GV, Sivolobova GF, Grazhdantseva AA, Akinfeeva LA, et al. Genotypic diversity of isolates and risk factors for hepatitis B virus infection in certain population groups of the Novosibirsk region. Infectious Diseases. 2004;**2**(3):39-44. (Russian)

[26] Netesova IG, Swenson PD, Osipova LP, Kisilev NN, Posukh OL, Cherepanova NS, et al. Markers of viral hepatitis B among south Altaians of the settlement Mendur-Sokkon (Atlai Republic). Subtyping of HBsAg of HBV isolates using a panel of monoclonal antibodies. Journal of Microbiology, Epidemiology and Immunobiology. 2001;**1**:29-33. (Russian)

[27] Netesova IG, Swenson PD, Osipova LP, Gubina MA, Posukh OL, Netesov SV. Determination of HBsAg subtypes in Western Siberian part of Russia. Journal of Medical Virology. 2003;**71**:183-187. DOI: 10.1002/jmv.10468

[28] Kruglov IV, Yashina TL, Tsvetova GV, Selyutina IA, Klimkin AY, Aksenova NF, et al. Spread of markers of hepatitis B and C and the etiological structure of the incidence of acute viral hepatitis in the population of Kuzbass and northwestern Kazakhstan. Journal of Microbiology, Epidemiology and Immunobiology. 1995;**6**:36-37

[29] Kuzin SN, Pavlov NN, Semenov SI, Krivoshapkin VG, Indeeva LD, Savvin RG, et al. The spread of viral hepatitis among various population groups in the republic of Sakha (Yakutia). Journal of Microbiology, Epidemiology and Immunobiology. 2004;**1**:18-22. (Russian)

[30] Zotova AV. Parenteral viral hepatitis in south Yakutia [thesis]. Moscow: Central Scientific Research Institute for Epidemiology of Rospotrebnadzor; 2010. (Russian)

[31] Kichatova VS, Lopatukhina MA, Potemkin IA, Asadi Mobarkhan FA, Isaeva OV, Chanyshev MD, et al. Epidemiology of viral hepatitis in the indigenous populations of the Arctic zone of the republic of Sakha (Yakutia). Microorganisms. 2024;**12**:464. DOI: 10.3390/microorganisms12030464

[32] Chulanov VP. Epidemiological and clinical significance of genetic heterogeneity of hepatitis A and B viruses [thesis]. Moscow: Central Scientific Research Institute for Epidemiolody of Rospotrebnadzor; 2013. (Russian). Available from: https://old.crie.ru/pdf/avtoref1(chulanov).pdf

[33] Ohba K, Mizokami M, Kato T, Ueda R, Gurtsenvitch V, Senyuta N, et al. Seroprevalence of hepatitis B virus, hepatitis C virus and GB virus-C

infection in Siberia. Epidemiology and Infection. 1999;**122**(1):139-143. DOI: 10.1017/S0950268898001940

[34] Schillie S, Vellozzi C, Reingold A, Harris A, Haber P, Ward JW, et al. Prevention of hepatitis B virus infection in the United States: Recommendations of the advisory committee on immunization practices. MMWR - Recommendations and Reports. 2018;**67** (RR-1):1-31. DOI: 10.15585/mmwr.rr6701a1

[35] Federal Center for Hygiene and Epidemiology of Rospotrebnadzor. Guidelines: Epidemiological Surveillance of Hepatitis B. Moscow: Federal Center for Hygiene and Epidemiology of Rospotrebnadzor; 2010. 47 p. (Russian). Available from: https://www.rospotrebnadzor.ru/documents/details.php?ELEMENT_ID=4825

[36] Ye X, Li T, Zhang R, Liu H, Zeng J, Hong W, et al. Comprehensive analysis of hepatitis B virus infections in blood donors in southern China that are surface antigen positive but nucleic acid testing negative. Transfusion. 2020; **60**(7):1476-1482. DOI: 10.1111/trf.15824

[37] Manuylov V, Chulanov V, Bezuglova L, Chub E, Karlsen A, Kyuregyan K, et al. Genetic diversity and possible origins of the hepatitis B virus in Siberian natives. Viruses. 2022;**14**:2465. DOI: 10.3390/v14112465

[38] Federal Service for Supervision of Rights Protection consumers and well-being person. State Report on the State of Sanitary and Epidemiological Well-Being of the Population in the Russian Federation in 2021. Moscow: Federal Service for Supervision of Rights Protection consumers and well-being person; 2022. 340 p. (Russian). Available from: https://rospotrebnadzor.ru/documents/details.php?ELEMENT_ID=18266 https://rospotrebnadzor.ru/documents/details.php?ELEMENT_ID=21796

[39] Mikhailov MI, Gomberg MA, Dolzhanskaya NA, Koubanova AA. Significance of sexual route of transmission of hepatitis B and C in Russia. International Journal of STD & AIDS. 2002;**13**(Suppl 2):9-11. DOI: 10.1258/095646202762226083

[40] Pokrovsky VI, Totolyan AA. Editors. Viral Hepatitis in the Russian Federation: An Analytical Review. Issue 11. St. Petersburg: FBUN NIIEM named after Pasteur; 2018. 112 p. (Russian). Available from: https://www.pasteurorg.ru/files/materials/photo/2020/VirHep2018.pdf

[41] Kuzin SN, Semenenko TA, Klushkina VV, Vlasenko NV, Churilova NS, Panasyuk YV, et al. Herd immunity to hepatitis B in the Russian Federation in 2017–2019. Epidemiology and Vaccinal Prevention. 2022;**21**(2): 29-37. (Russian). DOI: 10.31631/2073-3046-2022-21-2-29-37

[42] Moiseeva KE, Alekseeva AV. Main reasons for vaccination refusals. Social Aspects of Population Health (serial online). 2019;**65**(5):9. (Russian). DOI: 10.21045/2071-5021-2019-65-5-9

Chapter 3

A Case of Severe Acute Hepatitis B Virus Infection

Jasminka Petrović, Danijel Bijedić, Alma Trnačević, Azra Gutić Hodžić, Humera Porobić-Jahić, Rahima Jahić and Dilista Piljić

Abstract

The fact that >257 million people suffer from chronic hepatitis B in the world aroused interest in presenting the case of an icteric patient with the symptoms of acute viral hepatitis and with the markers of hepatitis that initially left us in doubt. A 47-year-old woman suffering from malaise and fatigue, severe abdominal pain, icterus and vomiting was referred to a gastroenterologist, and due to suspicion of choledocholithiasis and verified cholelithiasis by a surgeon, the patient was admitted to the Clinic for Surgery. After ruling out the obstruction of the bile ducts, an infectious disease specialist was consulted, and the patient with HBsAg negative and anti HBcIgM antibody positive was transferred to the Clinic for Infectious Diseases. A molecular PCR DNA HBV was performed and viremia was confirmed; parenteral antibiotic therapy was continued. Considering the deterioration of biochemical liver tests and changes in the patient's mental status, antiviral therapy was introduced. Liver tests were gradually restored, the patient's clinical condition significantly improved, and after 48 days of hospital treatment, the patient was discharged. In this case, we remembered that HBsAg is an important marker in the detection of hepatitis B virus in patients, but it is not a decisive marker in acute hepatitis B, especially in the case of a more severe form of the disease.

Keywords: acute hepatitis B, severe form of disease, negative HBsAg, cholelithiasis, antiviral treatment

1. Introduction

Since the discovery of hepatitis B virus back in 1960, researchers have become familiar with eight different genotypes of the virus, which differ from each other in terms of nucleotide arrangements and have different geographical distribution. It is a virus that primary infects human hepatocytes; the immune system of an adult controls viral replication and expression, destroys DNA HBV and HBsAg from the circulation and responds by developing anti-HBc and anti-HBs antibodies. However, ccc DNA HBV remains in a small part of hepatocytes as a sign of past infection, and in some cases, it is reactivated, leading to hepatitis B reactivation ('flare up'). The HBsAg protein in the outer lipid bilayer represents the most important and the

IntechOpen

largest part of the virus and circled nucleocapsid protein HBcAg that we find only in the liver; the shorter form HBeAg is found in the serum [1]. The HB virus has a high frequency of mutation due to the absence of error correction control for the incorporation of wrong nucleotides in the replication process.

1.1 Clinical characteristics of acute and chronic hepatitis B virus infection

Hepatitis B virus infection (HBV) leads to a wide spectrum of liver disease: acute (including fulminant hepatic failure), chronic hepatitis, cirrhosis and hepatocellular carcinoma. The average incubation period is 75 days (range 30–180 days), most often 60–90 days. HBsAg and HBeAg are the first viral markers detected in serum. Within a few weeks of appearance of viral markers, serum alanine and aspartate aminotransferase (ALT, AST) levels begin to rise and jaundice may appear. HBeAg is usually cleared early, at the peak of clinical illness, whereas HBsAg and HBV DNA usually persist in the serum for the duration of clinical symptoms and are cleared with recovery.

The diagnosis of acute hepatitis B is made by the finding of the anti-HBcIgM antibody in serum, particularly in a patient with HBsAg and signs, symptoms or biochemical features of acute hepatitis [2]. Virological diagnosis is based by the detection of anti-HBcIgM antibody, HBsAg and DNA HBV in serum [3]. In some instances, HBsAg is cleared rapidly from the serum and anti-HBcIgM antibody is the only marker when the patient presents with hepatitis B. In the natural course of the disease, acute HBV infection will recover clinically and virologically including seroconversion to anti-HBs antibody without antiviral therapy in more than 95% of adults [4]. If the immunoclearance does not succeed in the complete control of HBV infection, leading to HBsAg clearance and anti-HBs seroconversion, HBV infection evolves into the low replicative phase or HBeAg negative chronic HBV [5].

HBV is a significant cause of fulminant hepatitis (FH); in Europe, there are between 5% and 18% cases; in Bangladesh and India, between 13 and 15% cases; and in Sudan, 22% cases [3]. FH linked with HBV mainly occurs in patients who have acute HBV infection, as well as in patients with reactivation (flare-up) of chronic HBV infection, either spontaneously or after the initiation or discontinuation of immunosuppressive therapy. Fulminant hepatitis appears more frequently as a hyperacute liver injury (LI): icterus and encephalopathy until the first 7 days of disease but also as an acute liver injury (ALI): icterus and encephalopathy until first 2 months of disease, then as subacute liver injury: icterus and encephalopathy >2 months of the beginning of the disease. Acute HBV infection and acute exacerbation of chronic HBV infection can cause acute liver failure (ALF) or FH with lower than 25% survival rate [6]. More serious ALI is defined with INR >1.5 without liver encephalopathy, while FH is defined with INR >1.5 and with the presence of liver encephalopathy without chronic or previous liver disease. Acute exacerbation (reactivation) of chronic HBV hepatitis can manifest in the form of FH due to its characteristics: rapid course of reactivation, multiorgan failure, cerebral oedema etc. Because of these progressive events, chronic HBV reactivation can be similar to FH, although the definition of FH is somewhat different.

Chronic hepatitis B infection has affected >257 million people in the world and caused an estimated 800,000 deaths from cirrhosis and HCC. In >80% of the cases of acute HBV the infection ends with healing and loss of HBsAg, but due to persistent viremia, there is a possibility for chronic infection. Chronic HBV is defined by the presence of detectable HBsAg in the blood or serum for longer than 6 months and encompasses a spectrum of disease [7].

Chronic HBV reactivation is defined by the increase of DNA HBV > 1 logarithm in patients who have already had positive DNA HBV or by the reappearance of DNA HBV in patients with previously negative DNA HBV.

In the early stage of HBV infection, the virus does not stimulate the immune system. In the later stage of infection, the cellular immunity reacts, so do effector cells and humoral immunity with the appearance of antibodies. HBV elimination starts a few weeks before the beginning of the disease by non-cytolytic mechanisms of T0cell immunity. Later, the cytolytic immune response causes symptoms of hepatitis. Numerous CD8 cytolytic cells are present in the liver in this phase; they react with multiple Ag epitopes and eliminate the virus by destroying infected cells. The rise in arginase levels suppresses the activated function of CD8 T cells and has the aim to limit the amount of liver cells that will be damaged in acute hepatitis B [8]. Furthermore, soluble Fas antigens are present in high levels in patients with this form of the disease, which suggests that apoptosis is a principal mechanism in FH [9]. Therefore, the absence or presence of the virus at very low levels at the time when the disease manifests itself is an argument against antiviral therapy for acute HBV hepatitis [4].

The severity of acute HBV infection is also in relation to the characteristics of the virus itself, such as D genotype, viral D coinfection or viral mutations (precore mutation) in HBV virus [9, 10]. The principal cause of acute reactivation of chronic HBV infection is rapid increase of HBV replication from low levels that reflects on positive or high values of DNA HBV, anti HBcIgM antibody and HBeAg. During this phase, aminotransferase levels rise, jaundice appears and HBV viremia starts to fall. An increase of T cell response against HBeAg and HBcAg occurs in the early stage of exacerbation (acute flare-up) and declines after recovery from acute exacerbation and HBeAg seroconversion [11]. Spontaneous flare-up mainly appears in HBeAg-negative patients.

Anti-HBcIgM antibody is strongly positive in acute HBV infection, and it demonstrates a higher level, while the lower levels more often reflect reactivation [12]. HBsAg is an unreliable diagnostic marker of severe acute HBV with liver failure, the reason it becomes undetectable. In a study by Dao et al., HBsAg was positive in 20% of cases because of massive destroyed infected hepatocytes in severe acute HBV [13, 14]. However, DNA HBV has a lower level in serious liver injuries in acute HBV in relation to chronic HBV reactivation, such as HBeAg. So, low-level or undetectable anti-HBcIgM antibody and high-level HBV viremia could primary point to the reactivation of chronic HBV then to acute HBV in severe HBV hepatitis [14, 15].

2. Case report

The indication for antiviral treatment in HBV reactivation is clear, although in severe ALI/FH linked to HBV infection, there is no clear consensus. In severe forms of HBV hepatitis, such as ALF/FH, the decision for or against the treatment could be rapid for the chance of spontaneous healing. For this reason, it is necessary to distinguish these two entities: acute HBV infection and HBV reactivation. Although their progressive course is similar, treatment strategies are different. The implementation of antiviral therapy in the case of severe acute HBV hepatitis could shorten the disease duration, reduce the risk progression to FH and reduce the graft infection risk in the case of the need for liver transplantation. However, due to rapid reduction of HBV replication when HBV viremia is low, there is no clear consensus of antiviral therapy. On the contrary, in chronic HBV reactivation and high HBV replication antiviral therapy with nucleoside/nucleotide analogues is justified.

The aim of this article was to present a severe form of HBV infection and specific treatment for the disease in the case of a 47-year-old patient with clear icterus, abdominal pain accompanied with vomitus and malaise who was transferred from the Clinic for Surgery to the Infectious Diseases Clinic in Tuzla on 20 December 2023. We retrogradely analysed clinical characteristics of the patient on admission and outcomes: symptoms, biochemistry, microbiological and radiological results obtained from the electronic medical records and follow-up documents. The authors used the Microsoft Excel programme, while the calculation value change over time was done by the chain index. The diagnosis of acute HBV is based on the detection of DNA HBV and anti-HBcIgM antibody in serum, but severe acute HBV with the fulminant form of disease we define as coagulopathy (INR $\geq$1,5), jaundice (total bilirubin in serum $\geq$171 μmol/l) and with encephalopathy (any kind of consciousness disorder) within 4 weeks without data of prior liver disease.

3 to 4 days before the onset of symptoms, the patient had lost her appetite and felt malaise. The stool was regular, and urine was dark yellow coloured. Due to the suspicion of choledocholithiasis, the patient was examined by an internist gastroenterologist; abdominal CT was performed, which revealed two calculus in the infundibulum of gall bladder and the suspicion of gall blader mucosal dissection, so the patient was hospitalised in the Clinic for Surgery. Viral hepatitis markers were done, and anti-HBc IgM antibody was positive (3.57), HBsAg and HBeAg were negative, anti-HBe antibody was positive and anti-HBs antibody was also positive (45.8 IU/ml). Anti-HAV IgM antibody and anti-HCV antibody were negative. Aminotransferase was >20 times elevated compared to ULN, and total bilirubin nine times with higher values of direct bilirubin; leucocyte and CRP were normal. After the abdominal ultrasound, the rupture of gall bladder and choledocholithiasis were eliminated; an infectiologist was consulted and the patient was transferred to the Clinic for Infectious Diseases. The previously requested PCR DNA HBV was positive (1.15×10^4 IU/ml) though PCR RNA HCV was negative.

In the Clinic for Infectious Diseases, abdominal ultrasound described hepatomegaly (MCL 163.8 mm), hypoechoic liver parenchyma and spleen with rounded edges. A small amount of ascites was present. On the second day in the Clinic for Infectious Diseases, urea was low (1.8) with Plt 73, with increased bilirubin and ammonium in serum, coagulopathy. Due to persistent nausea, vomiting and confusion noticed the next day, Pantoprasol ampoules and Hepamerz pulvis, 2 × 3 g were prescribed. On the sixth day, the patient was occasionally somnolent and carbohydrate diet was introduced. On the 15th day of hospitalisation in the Clinic for Infectious Diseases, the value of total bilirubin in serum was 333.5, direct 170.9; indirect 162.6; serological tests for leptospirosis, Q fever, brucellae, haemorrhagic fever, markers for autoimmune hepatitis, antibodies IgM for herpes simplex virus, *Toxoplasma gondii*, Cytomegalovirus and Rubella virus were negative; antibodies IgM and IgG for herpes simplex virus type 2 were positive. The patient became agitated, refused the treatment as well as adequate oral intake of fluid and food. Voluntarily, without the knowledge of the hospital staff, she left the hospital, but with the involvement of the health care workers and her family, she came back after 24 hours and the treatment continued.

In the following days, an abdominal CT contrast scan was performed and hepatomegaly (240 mm in MCL) was described with periportal oedema, thickened gall bladder wall and several stones in the lumen; portal vein measured 14 mm; slight splenomegaly and microcalculi in the right rein were present. The abdominal pain was worsened and was associated with vomitus and higher aminotransferase levels. Lamivudine tablets 100 mg, 1 x 1 per day was available in the hospital pharmacy and was introduced on the 17th day of hospitalisation. Bilirubin had increased (378.4), AST: 2416; ALT 1390; NH3:

DOI: http://dx.doi.org/10.5772/intechopen.1009099

	1 day	2 days	15 days	17 days	23 days	31 days	41 days	50 days
				1 day Lam	1 day TDF	8 day TDF		Discharge
Le ($\times 10^9$/L)	4.87	5.2	5.9	6.95				
Hb (g/L)	120	109	113	121				
Plt ($\times 10^9$/L)	102	73	234	251				
CRP (mg/L)	21	16.2	9.0	10.5		9.8		
glucose (mmol/L)	5.2	4.2	4.5	4.5	4.7	7.0	4.4	
Urea (mmol/L)	2.6	1.8	5.8	5.2	6.1	6.4	3.2	
Creatinine (µmol/L)	78	80		68	78	77		
Bilirubin tot (µmol/L)	171	231.1	333.5	378.4	437.0	388.0	423.8	153.4
AST (U/L)	1066	1629	1638	2416	1206	633	258	91
ALT (U/L)	1996	1440	736	1390	748	307	174	49
NH3 (mmol/L)	17	44	37	50	42	33	48	
GGT (U/L)	40	40	76			55		
Tot protein (g/L)	48	64	66	60	74	72		
Albumin (g/L)	22	30	29	26	34	32		
PV (s)	15.6	16.9	16.8	14.2	16.2	16.4	13.7	13.0
INR	1.5	1.6	1.6	1.3	1.5	1.6	1.3	1.2
a-PTT (s)	45.1	41.2	39.7	34.8	40.5			
ALP (U/L)	157	136	124				103	
A-FP (ng/ml	5.8			90.5			247.8	84.2
Feritin (µg/L)				1048				
PCR DNA HBV (IU/ml)		1.15×10^4		3.92×10^1			pos (<10)	
Anti-HBs At		45.8		61.60			284.0	
Anti-HBcIgM At	3.57		3.46				3.25	

Table 1.
Biochemical and microbiological characteristics during hospitalisation.

50; A-FP: 90.5; ferritin: 1048. The patient was subfebrile; in urine *Enterococcus faecalis* 10^5 was cultivated, so Ampicillin ampoules were introduced during 8 days. Aminotransferase and NH3 were gradually decreased, while the total bilirubin was increased to 430.5.

After 7 days of lamivudine treatment, total bilirubin was 437.0, direct 298.6 but indirect 138.4; aminotransferase decreased; AST: 1206; ALT 748; glucose: 4,7; albumin:34; PV:16,2; INR:1,5; a-PTT:40,5; IL6: 3,15. Due to high resistance, lamivudine was replaced by tenofovir, 245 mg, 1 tbl/day; the symptomatic and supportive therapy were continued. After a total of 7 days of antiviral treatment, the control PCR DNA HBV was decreased: 3.92×10^1 IU, anti-HBs antibody was 61.60. The value of bilirubin was variable, but still high value: 414.0. In the repeated urine Candida species were cultivated; soor has been detected so for the prevention of Candida infection progression Fluconazol pills 2 × 100 mg were introduced. On the control on 31th day of hospitalisation ALT: 307; AST: 633; total bilirubin: 388.0; NH3: 33. On the 41th hospitalisation day, anti-HBc IgM antibody: positive (3.25); anti-HBs antibody: 284.0 IU; HBsAg negative; immunoglobulin M, A and G were slightly elevated; A-FP: 247.8; thyroid hormones were normal. PCR DNA HBV was positive but <10 IU. On the 50th day of hospitalisation, total bilirubin was 153.4; AST: 91; ALT: 49; coagulation was normal and the patient was discharged home.

The biochemical and microbiological results are shown in **Table 1**.

In **Table 2** we present the evolution of some analysed parameter s over time during the hospitalisation.

ALT and AST progressively decreased related to the initial value before antiviral treatment; 2 weeks later, ALT decreased to 77.91%; AST to 55.56%; NH3 to 34%. Bilirubin total increased during the first week of antiviral treatment to 15.49%, but during 2 weeks (therapy with tenofovir), it decreased to 11.21%; from the initial value, it increased by 2.54%. PV (quick) and INR unexpectedly increased, which could be due to insufficient duration of antiviral treatment. Urea increased to 23.08% after 2 weeks of treatment with variable course during short hospital management of antiviral treatment.

On the first control realised 7 days after the discharge from the hospital, the patient regularly took therapy: tenofovir, silymarin, ursodeoxycholic acid and vitamin

	Before lamivudine	**7 days of lamivudine**	**7 days of tenofovir**	**Percentage change during 1.week (%)**	**Percentage change during 2.week (%)**	**Percentage change during 2 weeks (%)**
Bilirubin total	378.4	437.0	388.0	15.49	′−11.21	2.54
ALT	1390	748	307	′−46.19	′−58.96	′−77.91
AST	2416	1206	633	′−50.08	′−47.51	′−73.80
Glucose	4.5	4.7	7.0	4.44	48.94	55.56
Urea	5.2	6.1	6.4	17.31	4.92	23.08
NH3	50.0	42	33	′−16.0	′−21.43	′−34.0
PV (Quick)	14.2	16.2	16.4	14.08	1.23	15.49
INR	1.3	1.5	1.6	15.38	6.67	23.08

Table 2.
The evolution of biochemical analyses over time during hospitalisation.

B; occasionally she had mild pain in the right hipochondrium. In biochemistry: total bilirubin: 136; direct: 57.5; indirect: 78.5; ALT: 61 (36); AST 126 (30); amylase: 106; GGT: 54; cholesterol: 6.6; triglyceride: 4.4; Plt, glucose, urea were normal.

On the second control, 16 days after being discharged from the hospital, she declared that abdominal pain and vomitus were somewhat less frequent (after consummation of sweet food). She had no hepatomegaly and total bilirubin: 64 (21); AST: 54 (30); ALP: 146 (104).

After 7 weeks on the third control, the patient felt good. Total bilirubin, aminotransferase, GGT, platelets and glucose were normal; ALP: 146 (104); cholesterol: 6.2; triglyceride: 3.0.

4 months after the discharge anti-HBs antibody were 1000.0 IU with HBsAg negative (0.14) and PCR DNA HBV was positive (<10 IU). Liver enzymes were normal, cholesterol: 7,9; triglyceride: 3,1. The patient itself discontinued tenofovir due to hip pain after total 14 weeks of tenofovir treatment.

The biochemical and microbiological results after discharge are shown in **Table 3**.

	1 control	**2 control**	**3 control**	**4 control**
	5 days of discharge	**16 days of discharge**	**7 weeks of discharge**	**4 months of discharge**
Le ($\times 10^9$/L)	5.93	5.9	6.0	6.60
Hb (g/L)	138	129	136	135
Plt ($\times 10^9$/L)	186	168	173	161
CRP (mg/L)	7.26		1.07	
Glucose (mmol/L)	5.8	5.6	6.1	5.1
Urea (mmol/L)	4.0	4.2		7.0
Bilirubin tot (μmol/L)	136	64	15	7.0
Bilirubin dir (μmol/L)	57.5		4.9	
AST (U/L)	126	54	27	23
ALT (U/L)	61	29	14	15
GGT (U/L)	54	33	21	23
ALP (U/L)	133	146	146	
Tot protein (g/L)	84			69
Albumin (g/L)	36			
Cholesterol (mmol/L)	6.6		6.2	7.9
Triglyceride (mmol/L)	4.4		3.0	3.1
PCR DNAHBV (IU/ml)				pos(<10)
HBsAg				neg(0.14)
Anti-HBsAt				pos(1000)

Table 3.
Biochemical and microbiological tests after discharge.

3. Discussion

During acute exposition to virus HBV in adults, the immune system generally controls viral replication and expression and creates anti-HBc and anti-HBs antibodies. HBV elimination starts some weeks before the disease by T-cell-mediated reactions following cytolisa and symptoms of acute hepatitis. In acute hepatitis a great number of cytolitic CD8 T-cells are present in the liver [16]. However, less cccDNA rests in hepatocytes as a marker of past infection and in some cases is reactivated, causing HBV reactivation [17].

One of the decisive criteria for transferring the patient in the Clinic for Infectious Diseases was positive test of anti-HBcIgM antibody in the serum although HBsAg was negative; we were waiting for the result of DNA HBV by the PCR method. Anti-HBc antibody appears early in acute hepatitis B (4–10 weeks after the HBsAg appearance) as a result of HBcAg in hepatocyte's nuclei. In 5–6% of the cases of acute HBV, especially in fulminant hepatitis, anti-HBcIgM antibodies are detected without HBsAg detection [18], as described in our paper.

HBsAg was detected in serum 4–6 weeks after infection and disappeared from serum during 3–6 months. In 5–6% of patients with developed clinical symptoms, it disappeared earlier. That especially relates to the cases with fulminant HBV or HDV coinfection. Due to that reason, our patient was tested on PCR RNA HDV and the result was negative. Anti-HBe antibodies in circulation are detected some days or weeks after the HBeAg become negative, and they point to the reduction of infection. In this situation we could expect the resolution of biochemical analyses that had not happened in our case.

Considering that about 50% of patients with chr HBV have anti-HBcIgM positive [1], clinicians thought that low viremia and low titre of anti-HBcIgM antibody in the serum in the first days of hospitalisation were possible due to reactivation of the disease. Generally, the presence of IgM antibody in chronic HBV follows the replication of the virus, which in our case could not be proved due to the absence of HBeAg and the presence of anti-HBe antibody.

HBV infection can occur as occult infection (OBI) defined by the presence of replication competent DNA HBV (cccDNA in the liver) and/or DNA HBV in the blood of people who are negative on HBsAg [19]. Considering the presence of HBV-specific antibodies, occult HBV is divided into:

1. Seropositive OBI (anti-HBc and/or anti-HBs antibody positive)

2. Seronegative OBI (anti-HBc and anti-HBs negative)

Most of the authors confirm that DNA HBV appears only intermittently in the serum and then concentration is low. In seropositive OBI. HBsAg could become negative as a result of acute HBV resolution (couple of months from the HBsAg presence) or after the HBsAg positivity that lasts for decades (so = called "overt chronic HBV infection") with or without disease. Our patient had positive anti-HBcIgM, anti-HBe antibodies and biochemical features of acute hepatitis that did not correspond to occult HBV infection.

Dominant TH1 immunological response in acute HBV stimulates cell-mediated viral clearance, though TH2 immunological response in chronic HBV stimulates antibody production. Tests for anti-HBcIgM antibody must be quantitative though the value of >1:1000 indicates acute HBV with high inflammatory activities. In all other situations, concentrations are lower or nondetectable [16, 20]. In a study in Greece, anti-HBc IgM antibody of low molecular weight (7–8 S) is the most frequently found at HDV superinfection; the mortality was low. In contrast 19 S IgM anti HBc antibody were frequently recorded in spontaneous reactivation of chronic HBV, and death in that case was high [21]. In our laboratory, we could not determine the molecular weight of anti-HBcIgM antibody; our patient had increased values of immunoglobulin class A, M and G in the serum.

Also, in atypical course of acute HBV, in fulminant disease, DNA HBV and HBeAg become undetectable as fulminant hepatitis develops. Considering the occurrence of somnolence on the sixth day of hospitalisation in the Clinic for Infectious Diseases (it corresponded to the second degree of liver encephalopathy) there was the suspicion for the development of fulminant acute viral hepatitis including the lower value of Plt (71); increased PT (18.3; INR: 1.7), increased NH3 (44); decreased urea (1.8); glucose 4.5; WBC: 4.87 and decreased albumin (22). Total bilirubin was 252 with the tendency to increase. The patient was agitated, refused the therapy and suddenly unannounced left the hospital. Clinicians concluded that fulminant form of the disease was possible.

Anti-HBs antibody is generally detected in the reconvalescence phase of acute HBV. It appears when DNA HBV decreases or disappears, that is, several months after the onset of the disease, and persists for a long time.

In about 25% of cured acute hepatitis B, HBsAg disappears much faster, so the serum tested in the last phasis of acute disease can be HBsAg negative. That did not correspond to this case, where liver enzymes and general clinical conditions continuously worsened.

The mutant forms of the virus also influence the course of HBV hepatitis such as HBV-core mutant virus, so the clinicians were thinking about infection by mutant virus. In support of this, there were high values of aminotransferase and HBeAg negative but anti-HBe antibody positive marker and negative data of previous HBV infection. The viral mutation with or without the appearance of anti-HBe antibody happens because of incorrect incorporation of nucleotides during viral replication and inefficiency of reparation mechanisms that correct errors in the genome. Precore viral mutants escape immunological response in the host. On the other side, pre-S and S mutations in HBV genome with the exchange of amino acid sequences of HBsAg cause problems in the detection of mutant HBsAg, and false negative test result is found (commercial tests ignore modified HBsAg), but viral replication possibility exists in the presence of anti-HBs antibody, also. Also, circulated DNA HBV in these persons is comparable to that in HBsAg positive persons. Our patient also had HBsAg negative marker, viremia positive and anti-HBs antibody present in the serum. These facts with biochemical analyses that indicate clear liver injury that is seen in severe acute viral hepatitis could correspond to acute infection by mutant HB virus.

Studies of some authors have shown that in so-called nonreplicative phases of chronic HBV infection, spontaneous reactivation happens in 17–32% of cases (defined in most cases as reversion from HBeAg negative to HBeAg positive infection, and characterised by increase ALT and reappearance of HBV replication markers) [22]. It is significant that many adult HBeAg positive patients have mixed infection, which includes the presence of both type of virus: wild type and virus with so-called Core-promoter (CP) and/or, rarely, pre-core mutations (PC) that later change in dominance but not pure HBeAg negative disease [23]. Some authors also thought that acute HBV is pretty rare and that HBV reactivation most often presents as acute hepatitis B; it is clinically very hard to distinguish those two entities, so it is necessary to have a high degree of suspicion about this [24].

Typical condition of severe reactivation is icterus and very high values of ALT in patients with chronic HBV. In the cases where we know about previous HBV infection (chronic), diagnosis of acute exacerbation is easy. Moreover, in a country with middle and high endemicity, the possibility of HBV reactivation is high (27–70% from the possible acute HBV infection and can represent the first episode of HBV infection because it was previously asymptomatic) [16]. Patients with acute reactivation of chronic HBV can have positive anti-HBcIgM antibody such as in acute HBV, in which the values are pretty higher (>1:1000) [20]. Moreover, by follow-up of our patient after discharge, we verified the resolution of biochemical liver analyses to normal values 7 weeks later. Anti-HBs antibody was 284.0 10 days before discharge, which increased to 1000.0 mIU later, while the PCR DNA HBV was positive, <10 IU.

4. Conclusion

Normalisation of biochemical analyses with high values of anti-HBs antibody, the almost undetectable viremia in our patient treated by tenofovir disoproxil fumarat for only 14 weeks, corresponds much more to severe acute HBV with the fulminant form of the disease than the possibility of other forms of viral hepatitis B.

Conflict of interest

The authors declare no conflict of interest!

Author details

Jasminka Petrović*, Danijel Bijedić, Alma Trnačević, Azra Gutić Hodžić, Humera Porobić-Jahić, Rahima Jahić and Dilista Piljić
Department for Infectious Diseases, University Clinical Center, Tuzla, Bosnia and Herzegovina

*Address all correspondence to: jpetrovic2005@yahoo.com

References

[1] Delić D. Epidemiological and clinical charasteristics of chronic viral hepatitis. In: Đerić BJ, Marjanović M, editors. Chronic Viral Hepatitis. 1st ed. Beograd: Zavod za udžbenike; 2012. p. 38, 58-60. ISBN: 978-86-17-18028-5

[2] Liang TJ. Hepatitis B: The virus and disease. Hepatology. 2009;**49**(Suppl. 5): S13-S21

[3] Ichai P, Samuel D. Management of fulminant Hepatitis B. Current Infectious Disease Reports. 2019;**21**:25

[4] Anonymous. EASL clinical practice guidelines on the management of hepatitis B virus infection. Journal of Hepatology. 2017;**67**:370-398

[5] Brunetto MR. A new role for an old marker, HBsAg. Journal of Hepatology. 2010;**52**:475-477

[6] Ostapowitz G, Fontana RJ, Schdiodt FV, Larson A, Davern TJ, Han SH. Results of a prospective study of acute liver failure at 17 tertiary care centers in the United States. Annals of Internal Medicine. 2002;**137**(12):947-954

[7] Anonymous. WHO Guidelines for the Prevention, Diagnosis, Care and Treatment for People With Chronic Hepatitis B Infection. 2024. Available from: https://apps.who.int/iris/handle/10665/376353.

[8] Sandalova E, Laccabue D, Boni C, Watanabe T, Tan A, Zong HZ, et al. Increased levels of arginaze in patients with acute hepatitis B suppress antiviral T cells. Gastroenterology. 2012;**143**(1): 78-87 e3

[9] Rivero M, Crespo J, Fabrega E, Casont F, Mayorga M, Gomez-Fleitas M, et al. Apoptosis mediated by the Fas system in the fulminant hepatitis by hepatitis B virus. Journal of Viral Hepatitis. 2002;**9**(2):107-113

[10] Lettau LA, Mc Carthy JG, Smith MH, Hadler SC, Morse LJ, Ukena T, et al. Outbreaks of severe hepatitis dute to delta and hepatitis B viruses in parenteral drug abusers and their contacts. The New England Journal of Medicine. 1987;**317**(20):1256-1262

[11] Tsai SL, Chen PJ, Lai MY, Yang PM, Sung JL, Huang JH, et al. Acute egzacerbation of chronic type B hepatitis core and e antigens. Implications for hepatitis B e antigen seroconversion. The Journal of Clinical Investigation. 1992;**89**(1):87-96

[12] Wai CT, Fontana RJ, Polson J, Hussain M, Shakil AO, Han SH, et al. Clinical outcome and clinical characteristics of hepatitis B-related acute liver failure in the United States. Journal of Viral Hepatitis. 2005;**12**(2):192-198

[13] Ozasa A, Tanaka Y, Outo E, Sugiyama M, Kang JH, Hige S, et al. Influence of genotypes and precore mutations on fulminant or chronic outcome of acute hepatitis B virus infection. Hepatology. 2006;**44**(2):326-334

[14] Dao DY, Hynan LS, Yuan HJ, Sanders C, Balko J, Attar N, et al. Two distinct sybtipes of hepatitis B virus-related acute liver failure are separable by quantitative serum immunoglobulin M anti hepatitis B core antibody and hepatitis B virus DNA levels. Hepatology. 2012;**55**(3):676-684

[15] Han Y, Tang Q, Zhu W, Zhang X, You L. Clinical, biochemical,

immunological profiles of, and differential diagnosis between patients with acute hepatitis B and chronic hepatitis B with acute flare. Journal of Gastroenterology and Hepatology. 2008;**23**(11):1728-1733

[16] Kumar M, Jain S, Sharma BO, Sarin SK. Differentiating acute hepatitis B from the first episode symptomatic exacerbation of chronic hepatitis B. Digestive Diseases and Sciences. 2006;**51**(3):594-599

[17] Raimondo G, Allain JP, Brunetto MR, Buendia MA, Chen DS, Colombo M, et al. Statements from the Taormina expert meeting on occult hepatitis B virus infection. Journal of Hepatology. 2008;**49**(4):652-657

[18] Delić D, Nikolić P, Božić M. Structural characteristics of hepatitis B virus. In: Đerić BJ, Pijanović P, editors. Virusni hepatitisi. Beograd: Zavod za udžbenike i nastavna sredstva; 1998. pp. 45-59. ISBN: 86-17-06545-1

[19] Raimondo G, Locarnini S, Pollicino T, Levrero M, Zoulim F, Lok AS. Taormina workshop on occult HBV infection faculty members: Update of the statements on biology and clinical impact of occult hepatitis B virus infection. Journal of Hepatology. 2019;**71**(2):397-408

[20] Gerlich WH, Uy A, Lambrecht F. Cutoff leveles of immunoglobulin M antibody against viral core antigen for differention of acute, chronic and past hepatitis B virus infections. Journal of Clinical Microbiology. 1986;**24**(2):288-293

[21] Tassopoulos NC, Sjogren MH, Purcele RH. 19S and 7-8S forms of IgM antibody to hepatitis B core antigen in acute icteric hepatitis superimposed on hepatitis B surface antigen carriage. Infection. 1990;**18**(6):376-380

[22] Davis GL, Hoofnagle JH, Waggoner JG. Spontaneous reactivation of chronic hepatitis B virus infection. Gastroenterology. 1984;**86**(2):230-235

[23] Gish RG, Given BD, Lai CL, Locarnini SA, Lau JYN, Lewis DL, et al. Chronic hepatitis B: Virology, natural history, current management and a glimpse of future opportunities. Antiviral Research. 2015;**121**:47-58. DOI: 10.1016/2015.06.008

[24] Jindal A, Kumon M, Sarin SK. Management of acute hepatitis B and reactivation of hepatitis B. Liver International. 2013;**33**(Suppl. 1):1478-3223

Chapter 4

The Management of Patients with Hepatitis B after Liver Transplantation

Harputluoglu Murat and Dokmeci Abdulkadir

Abstract

The standard treatment to prevent hepatitis B virus (HBV) recurrence after liver transplantation in patients with chronic HBV infection is lifelong use of a potent antiviral agent with or without hepatitis B immunoglobulin (HBIG). Antiviral prophylaxis with a drug with a high barrier to resistance should be continued indefinitely after transplantation. Although HBIG doses and durations vary from center to center, they are generally adjusted according to the recipient's risk of HBV recurrence and concomitant diseases such as hepatocellular carcinoma (HCC) and hepatitis D virus (HDV). While HBIG-free or short-term HBIG plus antiviral treatment is possible in low-risk patients, the use of a combination of HBIG and antiviral for at least 1 year is common in high-risk patients. Long-term HBIG plus antiviral combinations should be used in patients with hepatocellular carcinoma and hepatitis D virus, and the decision to discontinue HBIG should be taken with great care only within the context of clinical studies.

Keywords: liver transplantation, hepatitis B, antiviral, hepatitis B, immunoglobulin

1. Introduction

Hepatitis B is a serious global health problem that can cause acute and chronic liver diseases. Based on hepatitis B surface antigen (HBsAg) positivity, an estimated 257.5 million people worldwide had a hepatitis B virus (HBV) infection in 2022 [1]. According to a study conducted in 2019, an estimated 555,000 deaths worldwide are due to HBV-related diseases [2]. The frequency of HBV in cirrhosis-related deaths worldwide in 2017 was 31.5% in men and 24% in women [3]. In 2019, HBV was the most common cause, accounting for 42% of all hepatocellular carcinoma (HCC) cases worldwide [4]. HBV causes 749,000 new cases of HCC and 692,000 HCC-related deaths each year [5]. Hepatitis B is one of the leading causes of acute liver failure (ALF) due to its high prevalence in the Asia-Pacific region, accounting for 20% of patients with ALF [6, 7]. The most common cause of acute-on-chronic liver failure (ACLF) in Asia is HBV [8].

In the West, 5–10% of liver transplantation cases are performed due to HBV-related liver diseases. However, in Asia, HBV is the main indication for transplantation [9]. Liver transplantation is performed in cases of ALF, ACLF, cirrhosis, and HCC caused by hepatitis B. At first, liver transplantation outcomes due to HBV were worse, and hepatitis B was one of the relative contraindications for liver transplantation [10, 11]. Post-transplant survival rates have been quite satisfactory after the use of antivirals and hepatitis B immunoglobulin. Survival rates have exceeded 85% at 1 year and 75% at 5 years [12, 13]. The purpose of this review is to provide healthcare providers with up-to-date information on the management of patients undergoing liver transplantation for hepatitis B.

2. Hepatitis B recurrence after liver transplantation

2.1 Definition

HBV recurrence after liver transplantation is defined as persistence or the reappearance of circulating HBsAg, with or without detectable HBV-DNA [14].

2.2 Consequences of hepatitis B recurrence

In the pre-prophylaxis era, HBV recurrence had a very negative impact on patient and graft survival. In one publication, average patient survival was reported as 12 months. Graft loss could occur in a short period of 6 weeks [11]. Although there are publications reporting that HBV recurrence after liver transplantation has negative effects, there are also publications reporting that it does not have a negative effect. Clinically evident HBV recurrence is only seen in patients with persistent HBV-DNA positivity. Additionally, in cases of HBV-DNA negativity in serum, persistence or reappearance of HBsAg positivity is not associated with graft hepatitis [9]. Lenci et al. reported that HBsAg positivity alone while under antiviral treatment may not have any negative effects on patient and graft survival [15]. Fung et al. reported that elastography results were not significantly different between patients with and without HBsAg seroclearance, and with HBsAg reappearance, associated with an overall 85% 9-year survival, without any graft loss or death due to HBV recurrence [16]. In another study, liver biopsy was performed in 36 patients while HBsAg was positive and HBV-DNA was negative, with no histological evidence of HBV infection found in any patient [17]. Contrary to these studies, Lerut et al. reported that 3 of 16 recurrent HBV patients developed fibrosing cholestatic hepatitis, and all patients died within the first year postoperatively [18]. All this data suggests that antiviral treatment is of vital importance, especially in the post-transplant period, and prevents adverse outcomes even if HBV recurrence occurs.

2.3 HBV recurrence risk

In the 2018 HBV guideline, the American association for study of liver disease (AASLD) divided patients into two groups based on factors to consider when choosing prophylaxis. In this guideline, high-risk recurrence patients included those with questionable adherence, drug resistance, high HBV-DNA at the time of LT, human immunodeficiency virus (HIV) coinfection, and hepatitis D virus (HDV) coinfection. Patients who were compliant, had no drug-resistant variants, and had undetectable or very low HBV-DNA values (<100 IU/mL) at the transplantation were considered low-risk according to this guideline [19]. In 2020, the European Liver and Intestine Transplantation Association (ELITA) divided patients into three groups regarding HBV recurrence risk [20]. These are as follows:

a. Patients with low virological risk: Patients with negative HBV-DNA before LT, regardless of the indication for LT.

b. Patients with high virological risk: Patients with positive HBV-DNA at LT and HBV-induced acute-on-chronic liver failure.

c. Special group: Patients with HDV coinfection: Although they have low virological risk, they deserve full prophylaxis. HCC: They have a higher virological risk in case of HCC recurrence. However, they do not need specific prophylaxis. Patients who are noncompliant with antiviral therapy after LT.

3. Prevention of hepatitis B recurrence

To prevent hepatitis B recurrence, the management of patients can be divided into two periods: pre-transplant and post-transplant.

3.1 Pre-transplant management

It is vital that all HBV patients on the pre-transplant waiting list have negative HBV-DNA levels to prevent relapse after transplantation. For this purpose, all HBV-DNA positive transplant candidates should be treated with high genetic barrier and potent antivirals such as entecavir (ETV), tenofovir disoproxil fumarate (TDF), or tenofovir alafenamide (TAF) [19, 21, 22].

When choosing an antiviral treatment, some points should be taken into consideration. These are the antivirals used before and the history of resistance to them, if any, and the presence of kidney and bone disease risk. Lamivudine and adefovir dipivoxil were previously very commonly used antiviral drugs. However, due to their high resistance rates, these drugs have been replaced by more powerful antivirals with lower resistance rates, such as ETV and TDF. Although TDF is an advantageous drug in terms of drug resistance, it is an antiviral that has the potential to negatively affect the kidneys and bones. ETV and TAF should be preferred in patients at risk of kidney and bone disease [23, 24]. TAF or TDF should be used in patients with a history of lamivudine resistance [19, 21]. Pre-transplant antiviral therapy is beneficial both in preventing post-transplant relapse and in improving liver function [25]. Since lactic acidosis has been reported in patients with a MELD score above 20 treated with ETV, close monitoring is recommended in such patients [25, 26].

3.2 Post-transplant management

The standard treatment to prevent HBV reinfection in patients with chronic HBV infection is lifelong use of a potent third-generation antiviral agent with or without hepatitis B immune globulin (HBIG) [27–30]. The combination of HBIG with a high genetic barrier antiviral has been reported to be better than the combination of HBIG plus lamivudine in terms of HBV recurrence rate (1 versus 6.1%, $p < 0.001$) [9, 27]. All major hepatology societies recommend this in their guidelines [19, 21, 22].

3.2.1 Antivirals

For the last 15 years, antivirals such as ETV and TDF, which have lower resistance rates and are more potent, have been used instead of lamivudine and adefovir, which have high resistance rates [31]. A systematic review reported that the combination of HBIG with ETV or TDF had better outcomes than the combination of HBIG and LAM in terms of the risk of HBV recurrence [32].

Since it is important to protect the bones and kidneys in transplant patients, TAF, which has similar efficacy to TDF but fewer effects on these organs, has found a place in treatment in recent years as an attractive drug [33]. ELITA reported that TAF can be used in treatment to protect kidney function in countries where the drug is available. However, since the evidence on TAF is still insufficient, the results of prospective long-term studies in LT patients with kidney failure and osteoporosis are awaited [20]. One study reported that TAF treatment had a more favorable renal safety profile compared to other antivirals [34]. Fung et al. reported that long-term entecavir monotherapy was highly effective in preventing HBV recurrence after liver transplantation. They also reported that ETV monotherapy was associated with a 92% sustained HBsAg seroclearance rate, 100% HBV-DNA negativity at 8 years, and an excellent survival rate of 85% at 9 years [16].

To prevent HBV reinfection, antiviral prophylaxis with a drug with a high barrier to resistance should be continued indefinitely after transplantation, even if the risk of reinfection is low. Antiviral doses are standard doses, but dose reduction should be considered in case of renal failure. AASLD recommends indefinite post-transplant antiviral therapy regardless of HBsAg and HBV-DNA levels [19]. The European Association for the Study of the Liver (EASL) HDV guideline published in 2024 recommends preferring ETV and TAF and avoiding TDF because giving TDF together with a calcineurin inhibitor increases the risk of nephrotoxicity [35]. Indeed, considering the available data and information, it seems more rational to prefer TAF rather than TDF in the post-transplant period.

3.2.2 HBIG

The mechanism of action of HBIG in preventing recurrence is not well known. HBIG is thought to act through multiple mechanisms. These mechanisms bind to circulating virions, blocking the HBV receptor on hepatocytes and promoting the lysis of infected cells via antibody-dependent cell-mediated cytotoxicity. HBIG monotherapy is not recommended because it causes high rates of HBV recurrence post-transplant [25]. Hepatitis B immunoglobulin is prepared by cold ethanol separation of human plasma containing high levels of hepatitis B surface antibodies. HBIG has a polyclonal IgG antibody structure against HBV, and its IgG subclass distribution is quite proportional to human plasma [36, 37]. Antiviral plus HBIG combination therapy reduces the risk of graft infection to less than 5% [25]. The major challenges in the HBIG treatment are high cost, parenteral administration, and the possibility of mutation in the "a" determinant region of the HBV surface gene. HBIG doses, routes of administration, post-LT administration frequencies, and durations vary greatly among transplant centers. There is currently no optimal prophylaxis protocol for HBIG therapy [31]. HBIG treatment can be divided into perioperative (first month) and postoperative (after first month).

3.2.2.1 HBIG treatment according to periods

3.2.2.1.1 Perioperative HBIG treatment

In the Turkish guideline published in 2021, intravenous (IV) 5000 and 10,000 IU HBIG treatment in the anhepatic phase is recommended for low-risk patients and high-risk patients, respectively, to prevent HBV recurrence [36]. In its recommendations published in 2020, ELITA recommended 10,000 IU IV HBIG to all (low and high risk) patients in the anhepatic phase [20]. The Spanish 2020 guideline recommends 1000–5000 IU HBIG IV in the anhepatic phase [38]. The EASL HDV guideline reported that most centers give 10,000 IU IV HBIG to patients with HDV in the anhepatic phase [35].

3.2.2.1.2 First 7 days

The recommendation of the Turkish HBIG guideline published in 2021 for the first 7 days is as follows. For the first 7 days after LT, HBIG should be given at a maximum daily dose of 2000 IU intravenously until HBsAg seroconversion. After the 7th day, HBsAg and anti-HBs titers are tested. If HBsAg is still positive, 2000 IU daily is administered for an additional 7 days [36]. ELITA recommends using 5000 IU/day IV HBIG for low-risk patients and 10,000 IU/day IV HBIG for high-risk patients for the first 7 days. ELITA reported that ideal anti-HBs titers (between 50 and 100 IU/L) can be achieved for more than 4 weeks with HBIG treatment given for 5–7 days postoperatively in low-risk patients. ELITA also recommends the use of HBIG to provide anti-HBs levels above 500 IU/L for up to the first 3 months in high-risk patients [20]. The AASLD 2018 HBV guideline recommends using nucleoside analog (NA) for 5–7 days or no HBIG in low-risk patients [19]. The 2020 Spanish guideline recommends 1000–2000 IU/day HBIG IV or IM in the first week [38]. The EASL HDV guideline recommends that patients with HDV receive 600–1000 IU IM/IV HBIG for 7 days postoperatively, followed by weekly HBIG for 3 weeks [35]. Since almost all guidelines recommend daily HBIG application for the first 7 days, this application is routinely applied in most centers.

3.2.2.1.3 First 1 month

ELITA recommends the use of on-demand HBIG after the first 7 days to provide ideal anti-HBS levels (50–100 IU/L for low risk, over 500 IU/L for high risk) according to the patient's risk group [20]. The recommendation of the Turkish HBIG guideline published in 2021 for the first month is as follows. If HBsAg seroconversion does not occur after 14 days after LT, HBIG can be given for a longer period. However, if HBsAg seroconversion does not occur despite long-term administration of HBIG, HBIG administration should be discontinued [36]. The Spanish guideline recommends giving 1000–2000 IU/week HBIG or an on-demand dose to maintain the anti-HBs titer >200 IU [38]. After the first 7 days, on-demand HBIG administration is frequent to provide ideal anti-HBs levels.

3.2.2.1.4 After 1 month

Most centers aim to maintain an anti-HBs titer of 100–500 IU/mL, depending on the recipient's risk level [39]. The Spanish guideline recommends giving 1000 IU/

month HBIG or an on-demand dose to maintain the anti-HBs titer >100 IU [38]. The maintenance HBIG recommendation in the Turkish HBIG guide is as follows. During follow-up, HBIG should be administered at monthly doses of 2000 IU, and anti-HBs titers should be above 50 IU/L [36]. ELITA recommends that after 1 month, HBIG may be withheld in patients at low risk of HBV recurrence, but antiviral monotherapy should be preferentially considered in the setting of prospective clinical trials or observational cohorts. ELITA recommends HBIG treatment for at least 1 year for high-risk patients, with anti-HBs levels >500 IU/L in the first 3 months, 100–250 IU/L between 3 and 6 months, and 50–100 IU/L after 6 months [20]. The EASL 2017 HBV guideline recommends short-term or HBIG-free antiviral combination therapy in low-risk patients but does not make a clear statement about the short term. In high-risk patients (HBeAg positive, with HCC, HDV/HIV coinfection, and HBV-DNA positive at the time of transplantation), lifelong HBIG + antiviral combination is recommended [21]. The AASLD 2018 HBV guideline also recommends HBIG and antiviral combination therapy in high-risk patients, such as HDV/HIV coinfection and in patients with treatment noncompliance, but does not specify a definitive statement regarding duration and dose [19]. For patients with HDV, the EASL HDV guideline recommends the following. After 6 months post-transplant, HBIG should be given in a dose that maintains anti-HBs serum levels >100 mIU/ml. Today, indefinite treatment with a combination of HBIG and a nucleoside analog (NA) is considered the gold standard. However, the number of publications reporting that HBIG treatment can be discontinued after 1–2 years is increasing. Further studies are needed to assess the safety of this approach [35].

3.2.2.2 Route of administration of HBIG

Hepatitis B immunoglobulin can be administered intravenously, intramuscularly, or subcutaneously. The route of administration should be decided after discussion with the patient, based on the availability and cost of the product [36]. A review found no association between the HBIG administration route and HBV recurrence after LT [27]. Hepatitis B immunoglobulin IM and SC administrations are safe and effective in maintaining adequate anti-HBs levels. Some side effects, such as pain at the injection site and bleeding in patients with coagulopathy, may be observed with SC administration. Switching from IV HBIG to SC HBIG significantly increases patient comfort [36]. The AASLD reported that SC or IM administration may be more convenient for patients undergoing maintenance therapy [19]. The Spanish guideline reported that SC HBIG treatment can be applied from the first week after LT (500 or 1000 IU per body weight) [38]. One study reported a recurrence rate of only 4% after 5 years when intramuscular HBIG injections were given in combination with lamivudine. Additionally, costs were reduced by up to 90% with this approach compared to intravenous HBIG regimens [40]. In a multicenter study of SC HBIG conducted in 2013, patient compliance was high, there was no HBV recurrence, no discontinuation of treatment due to side effects, and mean anti-HBs levels were above the 100 IU/L threshold [41]. Vatansever and colleagues reported that low-dose IM HBIG combined with an antiviral results in 4.5% and 5.8% of HBV recurrence in the first and third years after LT, respectively [42]. Since SC application allows patients to go to the hospital less frequently compared to the IV method during the maintenance period, it seems to be a more comfortable application method that can be discussed and applied with the patient.

4. Special considerations

4.1 HCC patients

The presence of HCC prior to LT has been associated with HBV recurrence after LT [43, 44]. It has been reported that HBV reinfection significantly reduces overall and HCC recurrence-free survival, and reducing viral reinfection with combination prophylaxis significantly increases survival in these patients [45]. Recipients with HBV recurrence had worse outcomes and higher tumor recurrence rates than those without. One study reported a significantly lower 5-year overall survival rate after liver transplantation in recipients with HBV recurrence than in those without (32.0% vs. 62.3%; $p < 0.01$) [46]. It has been reported that positive HBV-DNA at LT affects the mortality rate due to HBV recurrence in HBV/HCC patients [25, 47]. ELITA suggested that combined long-term HBV prophylaxis in HCC patients is excessive prophylaxis in 90% of patients and that this patient group should receive prophylactic treatment, considering their virological risk, as in non-HCC patients [20]. The ELITA recommendation does not seem appropriate for countries that perform living donor liver transplantation in patients beyond the Milan criteria (solitary tumor ≤5 cm or two or three nodules ≤3 cm), because in these countries, HCC recurrence rates are higher after living donor liver transplantation exceeding the Milan criteria, and preventing HBV recurrence in these patients is of vital importance. The Asian Pacific Association for the Study of Liver (APASL) 2015 HBV guideline recommended 1 year of HBIG+NA combination therapy for HCC patients [22]. The EASL 2017 HBV guideline recommends lifelong combination therapy with HBIG and antivirals in patients with HCC [21]. The APASL transplantation guideline published in 2024 recommends that the decision to discontinue HBIG in patients transplanted for HCC should be taken with great caution [48].

Rates of HCC recurrence post-LT in HBV patients have been reported to be around 10–15%. HCC recurrences are associated with poorer survival [49]. Patients with hepatitis B infection have a higher risk of local recurrence and distant metastasis [50]. Tumor progression is more rapid and aggressive in immunosuppressed patients post-LT. Corticosteroids are commonly used in post-transplant immunosuppression protocols. They stimulate viral replication by mechanisms such as binding to the glucocorticoid response enhancer region of the HBV genome. To reduce the likelihood of HCC recurrence in patients with HBV, it is recommended that these drugs be removed from immunosuppressive regimens as soon as possible [51, 52].

High HBV viral load ($>10^5$ copies/mL) before transplantation was reported to be associated with frequent HCC recurrence after transplantation. Many meta-analyses have reported that NAs can reduce the incidence of early recurrence and improve overall survival [53–58]. Chou reported that the HCC recurrence rate was significantly higher in patients with HBV recurrence than in patients without HBV recurrence (40% vs. 5.7%, $p < 0.001$) [59]. One of the indicators that tumor cells act as a viral reservoir for HBV is the detection of cccDNA in HCC cells [49, 60–62]. Combination therapy with immunoglobulin and NAs may reduce the rate of HCC recurrence. In a study, in patients who used long-term HBIG, annual HCC incidence was reported very low at 1.7% [63]. The HBV and HCC recurrences are closely related in patients who underwent transplantation due to HBV-associated HCC. Therefore, the HBV recurrence may be used as a predictor in forecasting the HCC recurrence in HBV-related HCC patients who underwent transplantation.

4.2 HDV/HIV patients

In patients with HDV, more than 70% of patients have evidence of intrahepatic HDV recurrence after transplantation. HDAg in the graft is usually associated with mild histological change unless there is active HBV recurrence [35, 64–66]. There is no specific prophylaxis for HDV reinfection. Therefore, the most logical way to prevent HDV reinfection is standard HBV prophylaxis with HBIG and antiviral therapy [35]. HDV is a virus that requires the presence of HBV. In patients with HIV and HDV coinfection, the combination of HBIG and NA therapy is necessary for prophylaxis because of the limited availability of salvage therapies when HBV recurs [19]. The APASL transplant guideline recommends that patients with HDV coinfection should receive a lifelong combination of HBIG and a potent NA [48]. ELITA and EASL HDV guidelines reported that indefinite antiviral and HBIG combination therapy remains the gold standard prophylaxis to prevent recurrence of HDV and that discontinuation of HBIG during treatment can only be considered in clinical trials [20, 35]. In light of this information, we can say that we need to closely follow the results of HBIG discontinuation studies in HDV patients.

To prevent HBV recurrence in patients with HBV-HIV coinfection, long-term HBIG administration combined with an antiviral is also recommended [36].

4.3 HBV + hepatitis C virus (HCV) coinfected patients

Coinfection is not uncommon due to shared routes of infection [67]. The interaction between HBV and HCV in coinfected individuals is still poorly understood [68]. Patients who are coinfected with HCV/HBV have faster progression to cirrhosis compared with monoinfected patients [69]. There are studies reporting better outcomes in coinfected transplant recipients [70, 71]. According to the European Liver transplant Registry (ELTR) database results published in 2013, 10-year patient survival rates in patients with HBV/HCV coinfection were lower than in patients with HBV mono-infection but higher than in patients with HCV mono-infection (61%, 68%, and 52%, respectively) [72]. There is almost no data on the post-transplant management of patients with HBV/HCV infection. However, the British Society for Transplantation reported in its HBV transplantation guideline published in 2018 that the presence of HCV infection did not affect the HBV antiviral protocol [47].

5. Treatment of HBV recurrence

According to the EASL 2015 transplantation guidelines, treatment of HBV recurrence is immediate initiation of entecavir or tenofovir [25]. In case of recurrence, HBIG is discontinued. In choosing antiviral therapy, risk factors such as previous antiviral resistance and kidney and bone disease should be taken into consideration. In patients resistant to LAM, TDF or TAF should be preferred depending on the risk of bone or kidney disease. If there is a risk of bone or kidney disease, ETV or TAF is used. The combination of ETV and TDF may be required in case of multidrug resistance [38].

6. Anti-HBc positive donor grafts

Using anti-HBc positive grafts in HBsAg-negative recipients has a potential for transmitting HBV infection. Recipients who are both anti-HBc and anti-HBs positive can safely receive anti-HBc positive liver transplantation without any post-transplant HBV prophylaxis because the probability of de novo HBV infection is very low (<2%) [25]. The AASLD HBV guideline recommends prophylactic treatment for all HBsAg-negative liver transplant recipients who receive an anti-HBc-positive donor graft [19]. But the ELITA 2020 guideline does not recommend prophylaxis if the recipient is both anti-HBc and anti-HBs positive. This guideline recommends prophylaxis with oral antivirals if either or both anti-HBc and anti-HBs are negative in the recipient [20]. Whether or not antiviral prophylaxis is indicated, all recipients of grafts from anti-HBc-positive donors should be followed with HBsAg and HBV-DNA tests every 3 months for the first year and every 6 months thereafter for life [38].

7. Vaccine

Although vaccination against HBV has been an attractive prophylactic approach, its efficacy has been controversial [37]. Success rates vary widely, ranging from 7 to 80% [73]. Further relevant studies in transplant recipients are needed

8. Conclusion

After transplantation, one of the powerful antivirals, such as ETV or TAF, should be given for life. In patients at low risk of HBV recurrence, short-term HBIG therapy should be given together with antivirals. Long-term HBIG treatment should be given to patients with HCC, especially those with a high risk of recurrence who underwent transplantation outside of Milan criteria. Long-term HBIG combination therapy should be given to patients with HDV, but the results of HBIG withdrawal studies in this patient group should also be closely monitored.

Author details

Harputluoglu Murat[1]* and Dokmeci Abdulkadir[2]

1 Department of Transplant Hepatology, Inonu University Medical Faculty Liver Transplant Institute, Malatya, Turkey

2 Department of Gastroenterology, Emeritus Professor from Ankara University Medical Faculty, Ankara, Turkey

*Address all correspondence to: mharputluoglu@hotmail.com

References

[1] Polaris Observatory Collaborators. Global prevalence, cascade of care, and prophylaxis coverage of hepatitis B in 2022: A modelling study. The Lancet Gastroenterology & Hepatology. 2023;**8**:879-907

[2] GBD Hepatitis B Collaborators. Global, regional, and national burden of hepatitis B, 1990-2019: A systematic analysis for the Global Burden of Disease Study 2019. The Lancet Gastroenterología y Hepatología. 2022;7:796-829

[3] Sepanlou SG, Safiri S, Bisignano C, et al. The global, regional, and national burden of cirrhosis by cause in 195 countries and territories, 1990-2017: A systematic analysis for the Global Burden of Disease Study 2017. The Lancet Gastroenterology & Hepatology. 2020;**5**:245-266

[4] Kim DY. Changing etiology and epidemiology of hepatocellular carcinoma: Asia and worldwide. Journal of Liver Cancer. 2024;**24**(1):62-70. DOI: 10.17998/jlc.2024.03.13

[5] Perz JF, Armstrong GL, Farrington LA, et al. The contributions of hepatitis B virus and hepatitis C virus infections to cirrhosis and primary liver cancer worldwide. Journal of Hepatology. 2006;**45**:529-538

[6] Patterson J, Hussey HS, Silal S, et al. Systematic review of the global epidemiology of viral-induced acute liver failure. BMJ Open. 2020;**10**:e037473

[7] Maiwall R, Kulkarni AV, Arab JP, Piano S. Acute liver failure. Lancet. 2024;**404**(10454):789-802. DOI: 10.1016/S0140-6736(24)00693-7

[8] Hernaez R, Li H, Moreau R, Coenraad MJ. Definition, diagnosis and epidemiology of acute-on-chronic liver failure. Liver International. 2025;**45**:e15670. DOI: 10.1111/liv.15670

[9] Roche B, Samuel D. HBV prophylaxis after liver transplantation: Close to the full success but at the price of long-term prophylaxis adapted to the risk of HBV recurrence. Hepatology International. 2023;**17**(5):1072-1074

[10] Todo S, Demetris AJ, Van Thiel D, et al. Orthotopic liver transplantation for patients with hepatitis B virus-related liver disease. Hepatology. 1991;**13**:619-626

[11] O'Grady JG et al. Hepatitis B virus reinfection after orthotopic liver transplantation. Journal of Hepatology. 1992;**14**:104-111

[12] Kim WR, Poterucha JJ, Kremers WK, et al. Outcome of liver transplantation for hepatitis B in the United States. Liver Transplantation. 2004;**10**:968

[13] Young K, Liu B, Bhuket T, et al. Long-term trends in chronic hepatitis B virus infection associated liver transplantation outcomes in the United States. Journal of Viral Hepatitis. 2017;**24**:789

[14] BTS Guideline Development Policy. 2021. Available from: https://bts.org.uk/wp-content/uploads/2021/05/BTS_Guideline_Development_Policy_2021.pdf

[15] Lenci I, Tisone G, Di Paolo D, Marcuccilli F, Tariciotti L, Ciotti M, et al. Safety of complete and sustained prophylaxis withdrawal in patients liver-transplanted for HBV-related cirrhosis at low risk of HBV recurrence. Journal of Hepatology. 2011;**55**(3):587-593. DOI: 10.1016/j.jhep.2010.12.036. Epub Jan 18 2011

[16] Fung J, Wong T, Chok K, Chan A, Cheung TT, Dai JW, et al. Long-term outcomes of entecavir monotherapy for chronic hepatitis B after liver transplantation: Results up to 8 years. Hepatology. 2017;**66**(4):1036-1044. DOI: 10.1002/hep.29191. Epub 2017 Aug 26

[17] Fung J, Lo R, Chan SC, Chok K, Wong T, Sharr W, et al. Outcomes including liver histology after liver transplantation for chronic hepatitis B using oral antiviral therapy alone. Liver Transplantation. 2015;**21**(12):1504-1510. DOI: 10.1002/lt.24218

[18] Lerut JP, Donataccio M, Ciccarelli O, Roggen F, Jamart J, Laterre PF, et al. Liver transplantation and HBsAg-positive postnecrotic cirrhosis: Adequate immunoprophylaxis and delta virus co-infection as the significant determinants of long-term prognosis. Journal of Hepatology. 1999;**30**(4):706-714. DOI: 10.1016/s0168-8278(99)80203-7

[19] Terrault NA, Lok ASF, McMahon BJ, Chang KM, Hwang JP, Jonas MM, et al. Update on prevention, diagnosis, and treatment of chronic hepatitis B: AASLD 2018 hepatitis B guidance. Hepatology. 2018;**67**(4):1560-1599. DOI: 10.1002/hep.29800

[20] Duvoux C, Belli LS, Fung J, Angelico M, Buti M, Coilly A, et al. 2020 position statement and recommendations of the European Liver and Intestine Transplantation Association (ELITA): Management of hepatitis B virus-related infection before and after liver transplantation. Alimentary Pharmacology & Therapeutics. 2021;**54**(5):583-605. DOI: 10.1111/apt.16374. Epub 2021 Jul 19

[21] EASL. Clinical practice guidelines on the management of hepatitis B virus infection. European Association for the Study of the Liver. Journal of Hepatology. 2017, 2017;**67**:370-398

[22] Sarin SK, Kumar M, Lau GK, Abbas Z, Chan HLY, Chen CJ, et al. Asian-Pacific clinical practice guidelines on the management of hepatitis B: A 2015 update. Hepatology International. 2016;**10**:1-98

[23] Chan HL, Fung S, Seto WK, Chuang WL, Chen CY, Kim HJ, et al. Tenofovir alafenamide versus tenofovir disoproxil fumarate for the treatment of patients with HBeAg-positive chronic hepatitis B virus infection: A randomised, double-blind, phase 3, non- inferiority trial. The Lancet Gastroenterology & Hepatology. 2016;**1**:185-195

[24] Buti M, Gane E, Seo WK, Chan HL, Chuang WL, Stepanova T, et al. Tenofovir alafenamide versus tenofovir disoproxil fumarate for the treatment of patients with HBeAg-negative chronic hepatitis B virus infection: A randomised, double-blind, phase 3, non-inferiority trial. The Lancet Gastroenterology & Hepatology. 2016;**1**:196-206

[25] European Association for the Study of the Liver. Electronic address: easloffice@easloffice.eu. EASL clinical practice guidelines: Liver transplantation. Journal of Hepatology. 2016;**64**(2):433-485. DOI: 10.1016/j.jhep.2015.10.006. Epub 2015 Nov 17

[26] Lange CM, Bojunga J, Hofmann WP, Wunder K, Mihm U, Zeuzem S, et al. Severe lactic acidosis during treatment of chronic hepatitis B with entecavir in patients with impaired liver function. Hepatology. 2009;**50**:2001-2006

[27] Cholongitas E, Goulis J, Akriviadis E, Papatheodoridis GV. Hepatitis B

immunoglobulin and/or nucleos(t) ide analogues for prophylaxis against hepatitis B recurrence after liver transplantation: A systematic review. Liver Transplantation. 2011;**17**:1176-1190

[28] Loomba R, Rowley AK, Wesley R, et al. Hepatitis B immunoglobulin and lamivudine improve hepatitis B-related outcomes after liver transplantation: Meta-analysis. Clinical Gastroenterology and Hepatology. 2008;**6**:696-700

[29] Rao W, Wu X, Xiu D. Lamivudine or lamivudine combined with hepatitis B immunoglobulin in prophylaxis of hepatitis B recurrence after liver transplantation: A meta-analysis. Transplant International. 2009;**22**:387-394

[30] Katz LH, Paul M, Guy DG, Tur-Kaspa R. Prevention of recurrent hepatitis B virus infection after liver transplantation: Hepatitis B immunoglobulin, antiviral drugs, or both? Systematic review and meta-analysis. Transplant Infectious Disease. 2010;**12**:292-308

[31] Cholongitas E, Goulis I, Antoniadis N, Fouzas I, Imvrios G, Papanikolaou V, et al. New nucleos(t) ide analogue monoprophylaxis after cessation of hepatitis B immunoglobulin is effective against hepatitis B recurrence. Transplant International. 2014;**27**:1022-1028

[32] Cholongitas E, Papatheodoridis GV. High genetic barrier nucleos(t) ide analogue(s) for prophylaxis from hepatitis B virus recurrence after liver transplantation: A systematic review. American Journal of Transplantation. 2013;**13**(2):353-362

[33] Childs-Kean LM, Egelund EF, Jourjy J. Tenofovir alafenamide for the treatment of chronic hepatitis B monoinfection. Pharmacotherapy. 2018;**38**:1051-1057

[34] Saab S, Song D, Challita YP, et al. Long-term outcomes with oral therapy in liver transplant recipients with hepatitis B. Clinical Transplantation. 2019;**33**(12):e13740

[35] European Association for the Study of the Liver. Electronic address: easloffice@easloffice.eu; European Association for the Study of the liver. EASL clinical practice guidelines on hepatitis delta virus. Journal of Hepatology. 2023;**79**(2):433-460. DOI: 10.1016/j.jhep.2023.05.001. Epub 2023 Jun 24

[36] Akarsu M, Onem S, Turan I, et al. Recommendations for hepatitis B immunoglobulin and antiviral prophylaxis against hepatitis B recurrence after liver transplantation. The Turkish Journal of Gastroenterology. 2021;**32**(9):712-719

[37] Orfanidou A, Papatheodoridis GV, Cholongitas E. Antiviral prophylaxis against hepatitis B recurrence after liver transplantation: Current concepts. Liver International. 2021;**41**(7):1448-1461

[38] Fernández I, Pascasio JM, Colmenero J. en nombre del grupo de trabajo para el VII consenso de la SETH; Autores participantes en el grupo de trabajo en representación de sus respectivos programas de trasplante hepático. Prophylaxis and treatment in liver transplantation. VII Consensus Document of the Spanish Society of Liver Transplantation. Gastroenterología y Hepatología. 2020;**43**(3):169-177. DOI: 10.1016/j.gastrohep.2019.11.005. Epub 2020 Feb 21

[39] Te H, Doucette K. Viral hepatitis: Guidelines by the American society of transplantation infectious disease

community of practice. Clinical Transplantation. 2019;**33**(9):e13514. DOI: 10.1111/ctr.13514. Epub 2019 Apr 14

[40] Gane EJ, Angus PW, Strasser S, Crawford DH, Ring J, Jeffrey GP, et al. Lamivudine plus low-dose hepatitis B immunoglobulin to prevent recurrent hepatitis B following liver transplantation. Gastroenterology. 2007;**132**:931-937

[41] Klein CG, Cicinnati V, Schmidt H, et al. Compliance and tolerability of subcutaneous hepatitis B immunoglobulin self-administration in liver transplant patients: A prospective, observational, multicenter study. Annals of Transplantation. 2013;**18**:677-684

[42] Vatansever S, Farajov R, Yilmaz HC, Zeytunlu M, Kilic M. The efficiency of low-dose hepatitis B immunoglobulin plus nucleos(t)ide analogs in preventing posttransplant hepatitis B virus recurrence. Turkish Journal of Medical Sciences. 2019;**49**(4):1019-1024

[43] Chauhan R, Lingala S, Gadiparthi C, et al. Reactivation of hepatitis B after liver transplantation: Current knowledge, molecular mechanisms and implications in management. World Journal of Hepatology. 2018;**10**(3):352-370

[44] Kiyici M, Yilmaz M, Akyildiz M, et al. Association between hepatitis B and hepatocellular carcinoma recurrence in patients undergoing liver transplantation. Transplantation Proceedings. 2008;**40**(5):1511-1517

[45] Zimmerman MA, Ghobrial RM, Tong MJ, Hiatt JR, Cameron AM, Busuttil RW, et al. Antiviral prophylaxis and recurrence of hepatocellular carcinoma following liver transplantation in patients with hepatitis B. Transplantation Proceedings. 2007;**39**:3276-3280

[46] Li H. Post-transplant HBV reactivation impacts the prognosis of patients with hepatitis B-related hepatocellular carcinoma: A dual-center retrospective cohort study in China. International Journal of Surgery. 2024;**110**:2263-2274

[47] Burra P, Germani G, Adam R, Karam V, Marzano A, Lampertico P, et al. Liver transplantation for HBV-related cirrhosis in Europe: An ELTR study on evolution and outcomes. Journal of Hepatology. 2013;**58**:287-296

[48] Kim DS, Yoon YI, Kim BK, Choudhury A, Kulkarni A, Park JY, et al. Asian Pacific Association for the Study of the liver clinical practice guidelines on liver transplantation. Hepatology International. 2024;**18**(2) 299-383. DOI: 10.1007/s12072-023-10629-3. Epub 2024 Feb 28

[49] Saab S. Recurrence of hepatocellular carcinoma and hepatitis B reinfection in hepatitis B surface antigen-positive patients after liver transplantation. Liver Transplantation. 2009;**15**:1525-1534

[50] Zhang SS. Liver transplantation outcomes of HBV-, HCV-, and alcohol-induced hepatocellular carcinoma in the United States: Analysis of national inpatient samples. Current Medical Science. 2023;**43**(3):520-525

[51] Lee JY, Kim YH, Yi NJ, Kim HS, Lee HS, Lee BK, et al. Impact of immunosuppressant therapy on early recurrence of hepatocellular carcinoma after liver transplantation. Clinical and Molecular Hepatology. 2014;**20**(2):192-203. DOI: 10.3350/cmh.2014.20.2.192. Epub 2014 Jun 30

[52] Ghaziani T, Sendi H, Shahraz S, Zamor P, Bonkovsky HL. Hepatitis B and liver transplantation: Molecular and clinical features that influence recurrence and outcome. World Journal of Gastroenterology. 2014;**20**:14142-14155

[53] Kuzuya T, Katano Y, Kumada T, Toyoda H, Nakano I, Hirooka Y, et al. Efficacy of antiviral therapy with lamivudine after initial treatment for hepatitis B virus-related hepatocellular carcinoma. Journal of Gastroenterology and Hepatology. 2007;**22**(11):1929-1935. DOI: 10.1111/j.1440-1746.2006.04707.x

[54] Li N, Lai EC, Shi J, Guo WX, Xue J, Huang B, et al. A comparative study of antiviral therapy after resection of hepatocellular carcinoma in the immune-active phase of hepatitis B virus infection. Annals of Surgical Oncology. 2010;**17**(1):179-185. DOI: 10.1245/s10434-009-0694-z. Epub 2009 Aug 29

[55] Zhang G, Yu X, Liu P, Huang X, Jiang X. Efficacy of nucleoside analogs for chronic hepatitis B virus-related hepatocellular carcinoma after curative treatment: A meta-analysis. Digestive Diseases and Sciences. 2018;**63**(12):3207-3219. DOI: 10.1007/s10620-018-5252-8. Epub 2018 Aug 23

[56] Chen XX, Cheng JW, Huang A, Zhang X, Wang J, Fan J, et al. The effect of antiviral therapy on patients with hepatitis B virus-related hepatocellular carcinoma after curative resection: A systematic review and meta-analysis. Oncotargets and Therapy. 2017;**10**:5363-5375. DOI: 10.2147/OTT.S150281

[57] Yuan P, Chen P, Qian Y. Evaluation of antiviral therapy performed after curative therapy in patients with HBV-related hepatocellular carcinoma: An updated meta-analysis. Canadian Journal of Gastroenterology & Hepatology. 2016;**2016**:5234969. DOI: 10.1155/2016/5234969. Epub 2016 Mar 10

[58] Liu GM, Huang XY, Shen SL, Hu WJ, Peng BG. Adjuvant antiviral therapy for hepatitis B virus-related hepatocellular carcinoma after curative treatment: A systematic review and meta-analysis. Hepatology Research. 2016;**46**:100-110

[59] Chou HS. Significance of hepatitis B recurrence in liver transplantation recipients. BioMed Research International. 2020;**2020**:2489526

[60] Roche B, Roque-Afonso AM, Nevens F, Samuel D. Rational basis for optimizing short and long-term hepatitis B virus prophylaxis post liver transplantation: Role of hepatitis B immune globulin. Transplantation. 2015;**99**(7):1321-1334. DOI: 10.1097/TP.0000000000000777

[61] Chun J, Kim W, Kim BG, Lee KL, Suh KS, Yi NJ, et al. High viremia, prolonged Lamivudine therapy and recurrent hepatocellular carcinoma predict posttransplant hepatitis B recurrence. American Journal of Transplantation. 2010;**10**(7):1649-1659. DOI: 10.1111/j.1600-6143.2010.03162.x

[62] Hu TH, Chen CL, Lin CC, Wang CC, Chiu KW, Yong CC, et al. Section 14. Combination of entecavir plus low-dose on-demand hepatitis B immunoglobulin is effective with very low hepatitis B recurrence after liver transplantation. Transplantation. 2014;**97**(Suppl. 8):S53-S59. DOI: 10.1097/01.tp.0000446278.43804.f9

[63] Beckebaum S, Herzer K, Bauhofer A, et al. Recurrence of hepatitis B infection in liver transplant patients receiving long-term hepatitis B immunoglobulin prophylaxis. Annals of Transplantation. 2018;**23**:789-801

[64] Ottobrelli A, Marzano A, Smedile A, Recchia S, Salizzoni M, Cornu C, et al. Patterns of hepatitis delta virus reinfection and disease in liver transplantation. Gastroenterology. 1991;**101**:1649-1655

[65] Lucey MR, Graham DM, Martin P, Di Bisceglie A, Rosenthal S, Waggoner JG, et al. Recurrence of hepatitis B and delta hepatitis after orthotopic liver transplantation. Gut. 1992;**33**:1390-1396

[66] David E, Rahier J, Pucci A, Camby P, Scevens M, Salizzoni M, et al. Recurrence of hepatitis D (delta) in liver transplants: Histopathological aspects. Gastroenterology. 1993;**104**:1122-1128

[67] Crockett SD, Keeffe EB. Natural history and treatment of hepatitis B virus and hepatitis C virus coinfection. Annals of Clinical Microbiology and Antimicrobials. 2005;**4**(13):2

[68] Abdelaal R, Yanny B, El Kabany M. HBV/HCV coinfection in the era of HCV-DAAs. Clinics in Liver Disease. 2019;**23**:463-472

[69] Kawagishi N, Suda G, Onozawa M, et al. Comparing the risk of hepatitis B virus reactivation between direct-acting antiviral therapies and interferon-based therapies for hepatitis C. Journal of Viral Hepatitis. 2017;**24**:1098-1106

[70] Waki K, Sugawara Y, Tamura S, et al. Outcome of liver transplantation for recipients with hepatitis B and hepatitis C virus coinfection: Analysis of the UNOS data. Transplantation. 2011;**92**:809-914

[71] Rifai K, Wedemeyer H, Rosenau J, et al. Longer survival of liver transplant recipients with hepatitis virus coinfections. Clinical Transplantation. 2007;**21**:258

[72] Guidelines for Hepatitis B & Solid Organ Transplantation (First edition). British Transplantation Society Guidelines [Internet]. 2018. Available from: https://bts.org.uk/wp-content/uploads/2018/03/BTS_HepB_Guidelines_FINAL_09.03.18.pdf [Accessed: March 9, 2018]

[73] Yoshizawa A, Yamashiki N, Ueda Y, et al. Long-term efficacy of hepatitis B vaccination as post-transplant prophylaxis in hepatitis B surface antigen (HBsAg) positive recipients and HBsAg negative recipients of anti-hepatitis B core positive grafts. Hepatology Research. 2016;**46**(6):541-551

Section 2

Hepatitis C

Chapter 5

Microbiome and Hepatitis C Virus

Naiera M. Helmy

Abstract

The progress of infectious diseases and the relationship between microbial communities is one of the main targets of multiple research studies over the last decade. This review illustrated the relationship between the microbiome and the hepatitis C virus during the disease stage until treatment. This review highlighted the alteration in the gut microbiome and its influence on disease progression. The design involved the studies screening the microbial communities in infected patients, especially in viral infection. As the drug efficacy and safety may also be involved during and after treatment, the review included studies on changes in the gut microbiome of patients after treatment. The future perspective of studying probiotics reflected the beneficial effects of probiotic bacteria and their potential use in reducing the side effects of HCV during infection and treatment.

Keywords: HCV, microbiome, gut microbiome, probiotics, prebiotics

1. Introduction

The specific ecosystem's microbial composition in addition to its functionality has been considered by many international associations. In October 2007, the National Institutes of Health released the Human Microbiome Project (HMP, www.Hmpdacc.org) which is a global project shared with scientists to achieve a number of aims (**Figure 1**) [1].

The microbiome includes bacteria, archaea, viruses, phages and fungi. The most prominent microbiota, mainly in terms of species is bacteria. Since bacteria preferred to live in communities called biofilm, this made them an advantage as a community living in a microbiome. The maximum number of studies between all microbiota is intestinal tract (gut). There are two reasons, that added to the priority of studying the gut microbiome. The first is an integral part of screening gut microbiota to host digestion and nutrition in addition to the generation of nutrients from non-accessible substrates such as xyloglucans found in onions and lettuce. The second is that the bacterial species of the gut microbiome comprises a greater diversity than microbiomes found in other body sites. The Human Microbiome Project and the metagenomic analysis database MetaHIT reported that the number of isolated bacterial species from human faeces is about 3000 isolates. The classification of species has been

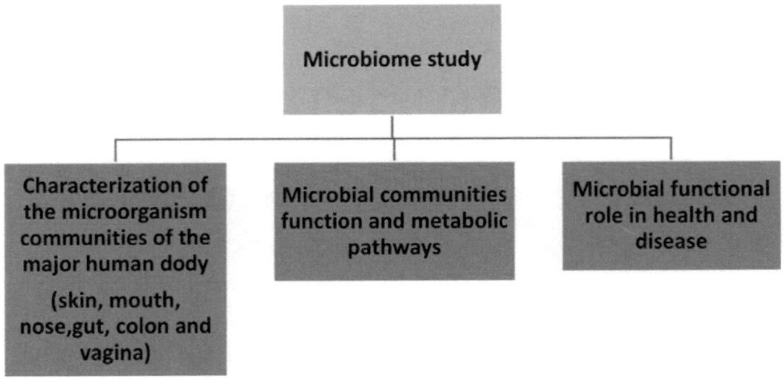

Figure 1.
Microbiome study aims throughout the human microbiome project.

categorised into 11 different phyla. Those classified with Proteobacteria, Firmicutes, Actinobacteria and Bacteroidetes cover over 90% of the gut microbiome [2–4].

Gut microbiota containing nonbacterial members were not getting great attention for a number of reasons; mostly their minimal abundance in the human gut microbiota and the shortage in the diagnostic tools required for assessment of the nonbacterial genome. Among the ignored members of human gut microbiota, there was an attraction to the composition and function of the so-called gut virome. The composition of human gut virome is bacteriophages as viruses belonging to bacteria, in addition to eukaryotic viruses with both DNA and RNA viral genomes. The minority of the human gut virome represented in eukaryotic viruses especially belonging to Picornavirus and Anellovirus genus detected in the faeces of healthy children. Studies also indicated that both bacterial microbiome and human gut virome go through substantial changes during the first 2 years of human life [5].

Hepatitis C virus (HCV) is a hepatotropic RNA virus. The virus progress can include acute and chronic hepatitis, through progressive liver damage. The cirrhosis, decompensated liver disease, and hepatocellular carcinoma are all signs of end-stage of HCV infection. HCV carriers were distinguished in about 2.5% of deceptively healthy individuals, and in about 24.9% of patients with liver diseases. About 35% of HCC cases were also HCV carriers [6]. As a public health threat, the World Health Organisation (WHO) to be started in 2016 and end called HCV for eradication by 2030. Even with some progress, there are about 57 million people infected with HCV in 2020, also 300,000 deaths occur each year reported with HCV infection [7]. For example, Egypt is one of the world countries showing the highest incidence of HCV infection, a lot of efforts have been directed to the targeted goal of WHO [8]. The overall plan in upcoming years includes the treatment with direct-acting antiviral (DAA) agents in addition to the prevention of new infections through a country-wide long-standing strategy [9].

The particles of HCV comprise a positive polarity RNA genome with 5′ and 3′ untranslated regions (UTR), also a long open reading frame encodes a polyprotein precursor of approximately 3000 amino acids. The translation process of the polyprotein starts with the ribosomal binding to the internal ribosome entry site (IRES) that spans most of the 5'-UTR in addition to the first 24–40 nucleotides from the region, which codes the core. The result is the production of a single precursor polyprotein being processed by cellular and viral proteases into 10 structural and non-structural proteins: core, E1, E2, p7, NS2, NS3, NS4A, NS4B, NS5A and NS5B. The core protein, forms the nucleocapsid. The envelope glycoproteins E1 and E2 constitute the virion's structural components. The assembly of non-structural proteins from NS3 to NS5B results in a membranous-web-associated HCV RNA replicase complex required in catalysing the amplification of the RNA genome of the virus. However, the independence of viral RNA replication on the structural proteins, all viral proteins are essential in the assembly and entrance of infectious virus particles [10].

Direct-acting antivirals cause inhibition of non-structural (NS) proteins necessary for the replication of HCV. There are three relevant drug classes: the first one is NS3/4A protease inhibitors ("-previr"; e.g., glecaprevir, grazoprevir) the second is the nucleotide analogue NS5B RNA-dependent RNA-polymerase (RdRp) inhibitors ("-buvir"; e.g., sofosbuvir) and the third is NS5A inhibitors ("-asvir"; e.g., pibrentasvir, velpatasvir) [11]. However, the complete eradication of HCV infection after DAA treatment is still indistinct through the persistence of some quantities of the virus after accomplishing a sustained virologic response (SVR) [12].

2. The development of gut microbiome discovery

The development of the discovery of gut microbiome and its relation to human health has been processed over a few decades ago. The analysis moved from technical challenges to analysing and discovery ability. The microbiome studies before were limited to culturing methods in which isolation of bacterial species was followed by sequencing of the bacterial 16S ribosomal RNA gene. In recent times, whole genome shotgun sequencing, and in another term metagenomic sequencing (MGS), has developed into a powerful method for studying microbial variations (**Figure 2**). There are approaches of (omics) such as metatranscriptomics, metametabolomics, metaproteomics and culturomics which added a deep link in the characterisation of distinct associated species and strains in addition to the relation between specific taxa and diseases [13].

As information from metagenomic DNA sequencing gives the perspective about the community's functional potential. This would provide the organism, the abundance and the biological processes but not necessarily, the specified gene transcribed under current conditions. The metatranscriptomic RNA sequencing as a culture-independent technology is overcoming this limitation. The collection of microbiome samples for metatranscriptomics should be preservative to RNA for sequencing regarding sensitivity, circumstances and timing of collection. In the process of data interpretation, the resulting metatranscriptomes must paired with metagenomes to avoid the changes in copy number of DNA (i.e., microbial growth) differentiation from changes in the transcriptional activity. The distinction in shotgun

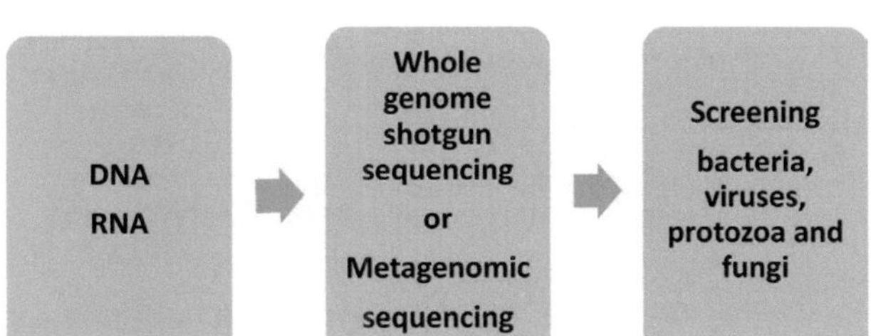

Figure 2.
Metagenomics application in screening DNA/RNA sample.

metatranscriptome is that the assimilated biological information is complementary to metagenome studies. Thus, comprising the detection of viral RNA and the quantification of the rare but function-based undetected genes in DNA-based metagenomic analysis. There are several steps for a single-microbe RNA-seq study, a representative metatranscriptomic study (**Figure 3**) [14].

3. Microbiome study and HCV

Several studies focused on the correlation between microbiome and infectious diseases. As the human body is continuously exposed to both resident and transient types of microbial cells and their by-products comprising toxic metabolites [15].

Shotgun metagenomic sequences led to strain identification through algorisms depending on either one of two techniques, the first is called single nucleotide variants (SNVs) in a community or among community members and reference genomes, and the second is the identification of variable regions such as gained or lost genomic elements [14]. The pathogenesis of hepatocellular carcinoma (HCC) affected by exposure of the liver to pathogen-associated molecular patterns (PAMPs) involves bacterial lipopolysaccharides (LPS), DNA, peptidoglycans and flagellin [16].

In screening study of gut microbiome between chronic hepatitis C virus and healthy individuals, the low bacterial diversity in persons with HCV infection was detected. The data showed a reduction in the order of Clostridiales and an increase in Streptococcus and Lactobacillus. The microbiota dysbiosis coordinated with the transient increase in Bacteroides and Enterobacteriaceae. Metagenomics' prediction of the microbial communities exhibited an increase in the gene of urease principally encoded by *viridans streptococci* throughout chronic hepatitis C progression. The

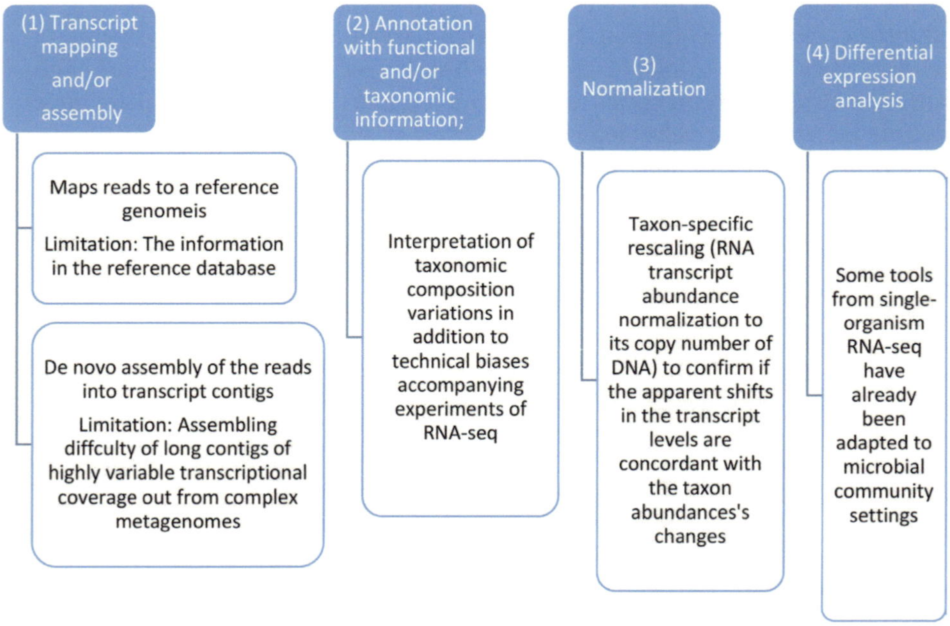

Figure 3.
General steps for a single-microbe RNA-seq study [14].

overgrowth of *viridans streptococci* could be the reason for hyperammonemia in chronic hepatitis and liver cirrhosis [17].

There are a number of factors causing the pathological effect on the liver through gut microbiota (**Figure 4**). The production and translocation of molecules such as peptidoglycans, lipopolysaccharides, DNA, lipoteichoic acid, indole-derivatives, bile acids and trimethylamine by microbiota to the liver and their interaction with liver immune cells has a great effect on liver function and alteration of the pathology of viral hepatitis [18].

The analysis of gut microbiome by 16S rRNA gene sequencing to the extracted DNA from stool samples of healthy individuals showed higher diversity than patients infected with HCV stage four. HCV patients were characterised with more abundance in phylum Bacteroidetes. Healthy individual samples showed higher abundance of Firmicutes, Proteobacteria and Actinobacteria. The analysis by genus-level indicated a higher abundance of Prevotella and Faecalibacterium in HCV patients while Ruminococcus and Clostridium were the most abundant in the healthy group. The Bacteroidetes's high abundance in HCV patients might be due to the overabundance of Prevotella. Bifidobacterium which is a probiotic genus was only detected in healthy individuals [19]. Prevotells might cause a reduction in short-chain acids that play a vital role in suspending the progression of HBV-related HCC [20, 21].

Studies on gut microbial dysbiosis throughout the progress of the hepatitis C virus and liver-related diseases are concerned widespread in the last few years. HCV and liver cirrhosis are the minor causes of gut bacterial alteration resulting in dysbiosis. A study aimed at the correlation between the gut bacterial community from individuals including healthy, liver cirrhotic and HCV patients. The collected stool samples were subjected to the 16 S rRNA using Illumina gene sequencing. Results indicated that HCV-infected patients showed higher *Enterobacteriaceae* and *Enterobacterial*, in addition to *Lactobacillus* and *Bacilli* when compared to liver-cirrhotic patient's sequencing data [22].

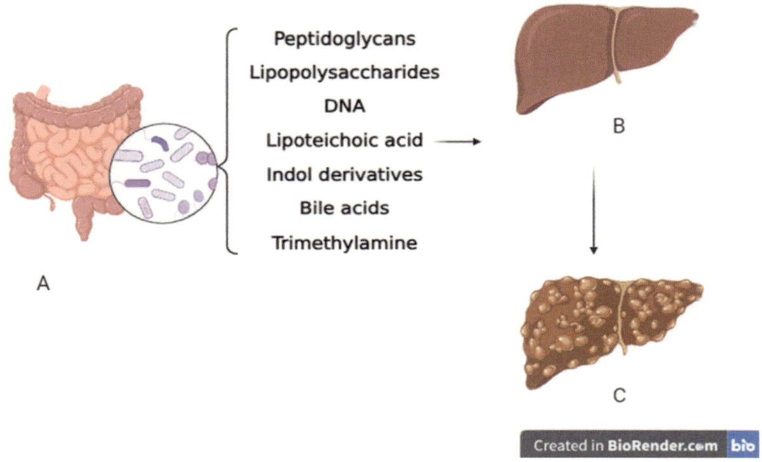

Figure 4.
Created with BioRender.com illustration of factors causing pathological liver conditions through gut microbiome. A: Gut microbiome causes release to peptidoglycans, lipopolysaccharides, DNA, lipoteichoic acid, indole-derivatives, bile acids and trimethylamine then translocated to B: Liver immune cells after interaction C: pathological effect on liver resulted.

HCV infection affects the metabolism of bile acid (BA) in the gut-liver axis through gut microbiota analysis from chronic hepatitis C patients (**Figure 5**). Gut microbiota significantly gets involved in the enterohepatic circulation through the co-metabolisation of BAs along with the liver. The study included a transcriptional analysis of the liver, mild CHC (fibrosis stages [F] 0–2), advanced CHC (F3–4) cases, and healthy individuals. The earlier disease stages of chronic hepatitis C patients exhibited BA profiles distinctive from healthy individuals, in which a significant reduction in faecal deoxycholic acid (DCA) and domination in lithocholic acid or ursodeoxycholic acid was detected. The correlation of the decrease in faecal DCA was found with the decrease in commensal Clostridiales in addition to an increase in oral lactobacillales. Impaired biosynthesis of cholic acid (CA) was detected by means of a decrease in the transcriptional level of the cytochrome P450 8B1 (CYP8B1) which is a key enzyme in the process of cholic acid biosynthesis. The decreases in faecal DCA and liver CYP8B1 were also detected in chimeric mice infected with HCV. The imbalance of bile acid biosynthesis performs the progression of the disease through the gut-microbiome-liver axis [23].

A study was directed to the identification of gut microbiota in distinguishing viral-related HCC (Viral-HCC) and non-hepatitis B-, non-hepatitis C-related HCC (NBNC-HCC). Stool samples from healthy controls and patients with Viral-HCC in addition to patients with NBNC-HCC. Faecal microbiota analysis was evaluated using 16S rRNA sequencing. The data established a decreased diversity and change in microbial composition of the HCC group compared to healthy controls. A significant abundance of *Faecalibacterium*, *Agathobacter* and *Coprococcus* was found in Viral-HCC patients, however, the five genera such as *Bacteroides*, *Streptococcus*, *Ruminococcus gnavus* group, *Parabacteroides* and *Erysipelatoclostridium* were higher in NBNC-HCC patients. Likened to Viral-HCC, the NBNC-HCC subgroup significantly showed a reduction in various short-chain fatty acid-producing bacteria, in addition to dropped faecal butyrate, however, higher plasma surrogate markers of microbial

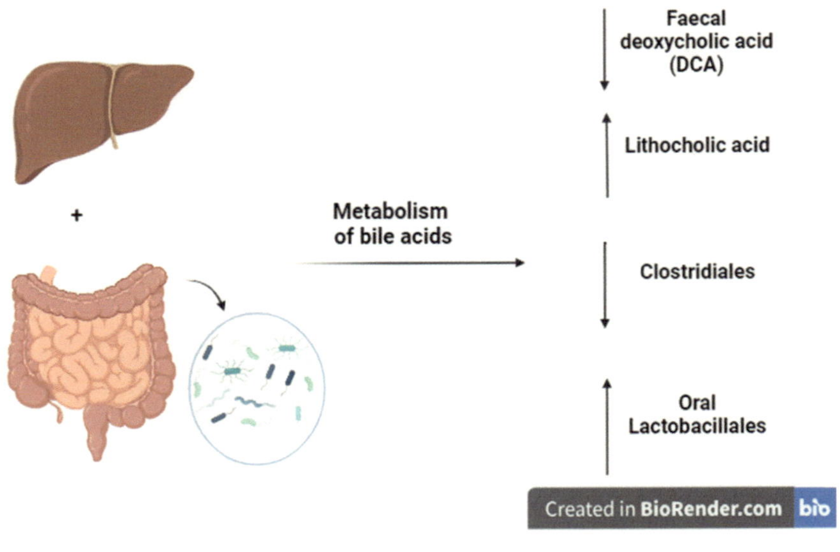

Figure 5.
Created with BioRender.com illustrates the effect of co-metabolism of gut microbiome and liver on bile acids. The reduction of faecal deoxycholic acid (DCA) and increase in lithocholic acid, in consequence to the decrease in Clostridiales and rise of oral lactobacillales.

translocation. The results showed that the distinction of gut dysbiosis depended on the etiological factors of HCC, which could be involved in hepatocarcinogenesis progress. The connection between gut dysbiosis and hepatocarcinogenesis could be used as a biomarker and a high-accuracy diagnostic tool to classify HCC subgroups. Microbiota-based signatures can exactly differentiate between infected Viral-HCC and NBNC-HCC [24].

Collected data from different studies performed on HCV using 16S rRNA gene sequence and metadata information from PubMed (https://pubmed.ncbi.nlm.nih.gov/) BioProject (https://www.ncbi.nlm.nih.gov/bioproject) was analysed to demonstrate the occurrence and progression of viral hepatitis and gut microbial diversity. The results demonstrated the decrease in gut microbial diversity and increased abundance of the genera *Butyricimonas*, *Escherichia-Shigella*, *Lactobacillus* and *Veillonella* which could be used as potential biomarkers for the risk of viral hepatitis. On the other hand, *Clostridia_UCG-014*, *Dorea*, *Monoglobus* and *Ruminococcus* genera are suspected as probiotics for HCV prevention and treatment. Vital bacterial upregulation might cause an increase in the production of metabolites from the gut microbiome such as tryptophan, lipopolysaccharides, fatty acids and lipids resulting in diverse roles in the activation of immune cells and inflammatory responses (**Figure 6**) [25]. The importance of tryptophan catabolism is in immune responses by protecting individuals from over-reactive immune reactions by inducting systemic immune tolerance and it is involved in HCV infection [26]. A necroinflammatory liver syndrome continues over inflammation by catabolism of tryptophan after 6 months of SVR in treated HIV/HCV-coinfected patients. Liver fibrosis in HIV/HCV coinfection would be in associated with dysfunction in immunity and tryptophan metabolism alterations [27]. The high level of lipopolysaccharides can stimulate the secretion of TNF and interleukin-6 (IL-6) as inflammatory cytokines cause the motivation of immune cells and lead to viral hepatitis progression [28]. Fatty acids play a diverse role in immune cells through inflammatory cell signalling pathways by cell surface or intracellular receptors [29]. The connection between lipid metabolism and the HCV life cycle is reflected through the enhancement of replication by modulation of lipid metabolism in infected host cells [30].

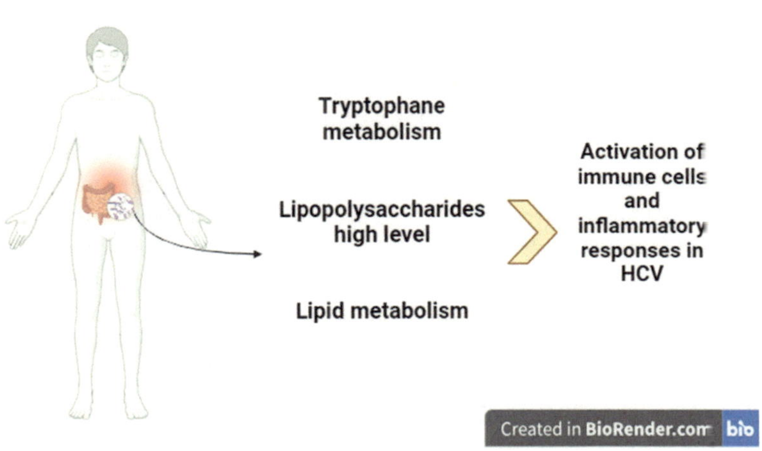

Figure 6.
Created with BioRender.com illustrates the effect of gut microbiome in the induction of immune cells through metabolic pathways of tryptophan, lipopolysaccharides, fatty acids, and lipids.

4. Gut microbiome and drug interactions

There are many researchers directed to the direct influence of the gut microbiome on the individual's response to a specific drug because of enzymatic transformation of drug's structure and alteration to its biological activity, biological availability, or toxicity. The whole phenomenon is called pharmacomicrobiomics [13].

5. Gut microbiome, antivirals and anti-HCV drugs

In the study for screening gut microbiome in patients with HCV cirrhotic with/without SVR treated using pegylated interferon and ribavirin after a median of 15 months and healthy control group. The serum and stool samples collected were analysed for IL-6, TNF-α and endotoxin in serum and stool microbiota was analysed using multi-tagged pyrosequencing. There was no significant difference in overall microbiota composition or within specific microbial families between the groups with/without SVR. This also includes the levels of IL-6, TNF-α and endotoxin. The two cirrhosis groups had significant dysbiosis when compared to healthy controls in addition to higher levels of endotoxin, IL-6 and TNF-α. In cirrhotics with/without SVR, microbial abundance of potentially pathogenic (*Enterobacteriaceae*) or lower beneficial families from Clostridiales XIV, *Lachnospiraceae* and *Ruminococcaceae* were detected when compared to healthy controls. Overall, Metastats and comparison of the cirrhosis dysbiosis ratios, there were not any significant differences between the cirrhotic patients with and without SVR. The results concluded that the eradication of HCV does not affect gut dysbiosis or systemic inflammation in cirrhotic patients [31].

The investigation of the contribution of curing hepatitis C virus (HCV) infection with DAA in reducing the progression of liver fibrosis and its influence on the gut-liver axis was studied through the gut microbiota composition, intestinal permeability, and inflammation before and after 1 year from treatment. The results indicated that the diversity of gut microbiota in cirrhotic patients was lower than that in healthy individuals. Thus, the overall composition of gut microbiota was significantly improved by the cure of HCV infection. After treatment, the abundance of pathogenic bacteria: *Enterobacteriaceae*, *Enterococcus* and *Staphylococcus* was decreased. There was an association between the composition of gut microbiota and the inflammatory profile and liver fibrosis markers. Even after a significant decrease in serum levels of cytokines and chemokines after treatment with DAA, there was no change in measures of intestinal permeability and inflammation [32].

Researchers demonstrated that gut microbes could influence drug efficacy and safety through the enzymatic transformation of drug structure and change in drug bioavailability, bioactivity or toxicity [13]. Both host and gut microbiota can metabolise the oral antiviral drug Brivudine (BRV) to bromovinyluracil (BVU). It was reported that the incubation of human and murine S9 liver fractions in addition to unfractionated faecal microbial communities with BRV resulted in stoichiometric conversion to BVU. This enzymatic transformation reaction was confirmed by both liver and microbiota with hepatic toxicity [33].

In order to study the short-term effects of DAA treatment on gut microbiota HCV patients. The HCV-infected and healthy individuals gut microbiome were evaluated before and after 3 months of the treatment. The results showed no dramatic changes in α-diversity in HCV infection, and there was not any recovery after HCV was negatively tested even if there was a complete restoration in lower fibrosis degrees. DAAs used for 3 months or in sustained viral response caused the changes in gut microbiota induced by HCV [34].

In another study on treatment-naive HCV microbiota. Increased diversity and abundance in samples were detected with *Prevotella*, *Succinivibrio*, *Catenibacterium*, *Megasphaera* and Ruminococcaceae. The low abundance of *Bacteroides*, *Dialister*, *Bilophila*, *Streptococcus*, *parabacteroides*, *Enterobacteriaceae*, *Erysipelotrichaceae*, *Rikenellaceae* and *Alistipes* was detected. The predicted functions of the metagenomic community displayed a reduction in carbohydrate and lipid metabolism in the microbiota of HCV accompanied by perturbations of amino acid metabolism [35].

In a pilot sub-study, variations in the composition of gut microbiota between patients after the successful treatment of hepatitis C virus (HCV) with glecaprevir/pibrentasvir (GLE/PIB) were observed before treatment and after 12 weeks. The patients infected with HCV genotypes 1, 2, 3, 4 and 5. There was not statistically significant differences in the gut microbiota diversity, however, there was a tendency to less richness over time [36].

A study investigated gut microbiome through 16 s rRNA analysed DNA extracted from stool samples of patients infected with HCV and HCV/HIV who received elbasvir-grazoprevir from a clinical trial. The analysis revealed less bacterial diversity in the patient group than in healthy controls. Microbial dysbiosis improvement was detected in responders completing sustained virological response through fibrosis stages which was absent in the case of non-responders. The alteration through the increase in beneficial bacteria and reduction in pathogenic bacteria was observed in responders. In the case of responders, the analysis showed the enrichment of *Parabacteroides* and *Subdoligranulum*. The reduction in *Eubacterium* was detected in both fibrosis and responders groups [37].

The examination of gut microbiota of targeted V3–4 region of 16S rRNA gene to clarify the changes in the microbiota before, and after (DAA) treatment of hepatitis C virus and 24 weeks after treatment ended. The data reflected that the gut microbial diversity did not show a significant difference between Pre-, End-of-treatment (EOT), and Post24. The comparison of gut microbiota in Pre-treatment and Post24 weeks after treatment showed a significant increase of *Ruminococcaceae* on family-based level and *Faecalibacterium* at the genus-based level. Furthermore, analysis at Post24 weeks of treatment, there is a significant increase in Bacillales at order-based level, *Bacillaceae* at family-based level and *Bacillus* at genus-based level. Moreover, there is an increased rate in the relative abundances of *Faecalibacterium* and *Bacillus* which further increased at Post24 when compared to Pre at EOT. There was a progressive decrease in genera *Bacteroides*, *Phascolarctobacterium* and *Fusobacterium* from the Pre to EOT to Post24. Whereas, the genera *Lachnospira*, *Faecalibacterium*, *Oscillospira* and *Akkermansia* increased [38].

The analysis of intestinal microbial community in patients who received DAA and achieved SVR and others without DAA. The V1-V2 region in the 16S ribosomal RNA gene from stool samples of patients was subjected to amplicon sequencing. The resulting data showed the changes in significantly increased relative abundances of two genera *Collinsella* spp. and *Bifidobacter* spp. in patients without liver cirrhosis. In addition, a non-significant decrease in the relative abundance of *Bifidobacter* spp. in patients with liver cirrhosis. At the baseline, only the relative abundance of *Senegalimassilia* spp. Among the genera that had higher relative abundances in patients with liver cirrhosis at SVR24/48: *Acidaminococcus* spp., *Eubacterium* spp. and *Lachnospiraceae* spp. Others exhibited lower relative abundances in patients with liver cirrhosis: *Citrobacter* spp., *Enterobacter* spp., *Enterococcus* spp., *Megasphaera* spp. and *Pseudomonas* spp. [39].

A cohort study on samples from adult patients confirmed HCV viremia prior to receiving DAA and after 12 weeks from complete treatment. The extracted bacterial DNA from stool samples was subjected to 16 s rRNA gene amplification and sequencing. Gut microbiome analysis showed a significant difference between HCV-infected patients with or without cirrhosis and uninfected controls. Analysis of the gut microbiome revealed that there are no significant changes in all patients attained viral eradication. However, the overall microbiome did not show significant variation shortly after HCV eradication. The analysis of the pre-treatment status and after 12 weeks of treatment showed enrichment in *Coriobacteriaceae*, *Staphylococcaceae*, *Peptostreptococcaceae* and *Succinivibrionaceae*. Also, the relative abundance of *Morganellaceae, Pasteurellaceae* and *Moraxellaceae* decreased after HCV clearance [40].

A study explored the role of the gut-liver axis in patients with chronic HCV-associated compensated liver disease (HCVi) through fibrosis severity by discovering the portal vein. In this study, blood samples from both peripheral and portal veins, liver biopsies and faeces were collected at two-time points and the re-evaluation was done approximately after 6 months of HCV elimination by means before and after SVR. Exactly, the achievement of SVR was reached after combination therapy with sofosbuvir and velpatasvir, oral inhibitors of viral replication. Analysis was performed through metabolomics on serum samples, RNA transcriptomics on both liver and faeces in addition to microbial 16S ribosomal RNA analysis on faeces. The results showed that *Bacteroides vulgatus* is the major active species on a transcription basis through the enhancement of hepatic transcription of the inflammatory pathways. This contributed to the functional predominant adverse effects of *B. vulgatus* on energy and immune homeostasis in patients of HCVi. On the other hand, inhibiting the effect of *B. vulgatus* in mediation of glycan degradation by manipulating diet or intestinal immunity suggests the early interventional therapy required to preserve the intestinal homeostasis occurrence in chronic liver disease [41].

In a study on gut microbiome on faecal samples from patients with HCV-related chronic liver disease. All patients were treated with DAAs (Paritaprevir-Ombitasvir-Ritonavir-Dasabuvir, Sofosbuvir-Ledipasvir, Sofosbuvir-Ribavirin, Sofosbuvir-Daclatasvir, Sofosbuvir-Velpatasvir) for 12 weeks achieved SVR. In all patients, there was a tendency to decrease pathogenic microbial species (i.e., Enterobacteriaceae). The analysis displayed that eradication of the virus through direct antiviral agents was related to the tendency to restore the heterogeneity of α-diversity besides the reduction in the percentage of pathogenic microorganisms, even if the patients with cirrhosis were less evident in this advantage [42].

A study illustrated the description of transcriptional alterations of the gut microbiome and liver after sustained virologic response on liver biopsy, portal blood (direct portal vein cannulation), peripheral blood and stool samples. HCV patients before and after 9 months from the 12 weeks of treatment with sofosbuvir/velpatasvir. The stool samples were used for RNA-seq and 16S rRNA metagenomics. The resulting data showed increased microbial products in the portal blood and liver after SVR. Investigation of gut microbiome after SVR indicated a differential increase in the genes encodes for the production of lipopolysaccharide from bacteria. As the decline in expression of the antiviral interferon pathway after SVR was predictable, there was an unpredicted decrease in the transcription of genes responsible for bacterial recognition and response. Thus, this was related to the increased level of microbial products [43].

In a study for the evaluation of the faecal microbiota before and after HCV treatment with DAA, faecal samples were collected before DAA treatment and 24 weeks after the treatment and healthy controls were concluded. The sequencing 16 S ribosomal RNA gene of stool samples was used to determine the taxonomic composition of the gut microbiota. The resulting data showed that the abundances of several bacterial taxa were different between the control and CHC patients. There is a significant more abundant of phyla Actinobacteria and Firmicutes in the CHC patients. The genera *Ruminococcaceae*, *Eubacterium*, *Agathobacter*, *Alistipes*, *Bifidobacterium* and *Klebsiella* were also enhanced in the patients of CHC. On the other hand, the phylum Bacteroidetes was more enriched in the control group also the only significantly more abundant is *Lachnoclostridium* genus. *Lactobacillus* was the only significantly raised in the CHC group when compared to the group of SVR24. Patients after treatment from HCV by DAA showed no significant alteration of the gut microbiota [44].

6. Other drug interactions with microbiome and HCV

The class of proton pump inhibitors, is associated with variations in the intestinal microbiota. A study aimed to clarify differences in the intestinal microbiota associated with proton pump inhibitors in patients with chronic hepatitis C. Analysis of the 16S rDNA gene in stool samples of patients with and without the treatment with proton pump inhibitors was established. The data investigation showed that the use of proton pump inhibitors was associated with significant alterations in the microbiota in patients infected with chronic hepatitis C. There is a significant increase in the relative abundance of *Streptococcus spp*., *Enterobacter spp*. and *Haemophilus spp*. reached in patients with the use of proton pump inhibitors [45].

7. Oral microbiome and HCV

There are more than 700 species or phylotypes of bacteria in the oral cavity, which contribute to health and disease [46]. The disturbance of microbial composition in oral microbiota could encourage the progress of many liver diseases [47].

A study indicated the role of the oral microbiome in hepatocellular carcinoma patients using 16S rRNA in extracted DNA from oral samples of HCC cases and other healthy controls. The positive abundance of Cyanobacteria associated with HCC. The Cyanobacterial genes positive association with HCC were particular to taxa-producing microcystin which is a hepatotoxic tumour promotor in addition to other genes identified to be upregulated with the exposure to microcystin [48].

A case-control preliminary study on HCV patients, patients reached viral clearance after DAA treatment and healthy individuals. The 16S rRNA was sequenced from a buccal swab. The results referred to the significant distinct bacterial community in the oral microbiome of patients with chronic HCV compared to healthy controls. The oral microbiome of HCV patients was characterised by a high diversity and abundance of pathogenic species, which is similar to that of the oral lichen planus patients. However, the shift in oral microbiome after the treatment with DAA to a community was indicative to be partially similar to both diseased and healthy ones [49].

The transmission of HCV *via* the oral cavity reflected the importance of determining the virulence factor homologues of the oral viromes in using the concept of viral reserving pathogenic gene functions [50]. The effect of antiviral therapy comprising interferon-alpha (IFN-alpha) with or without ribavirin on oral lichen planus (OLP) has been distinguished. After HCV treatment, some patients face an enhancement in OLP lesions [51]. Studies have strengthened the concept that the improvement of OLP clinical outcomes was investigated with modern DAA treatment in HCV-infected patients. This confirmation sustained the suggestion that HCV successful antiviral therapy directed improvements in the symptoms of OLP [52].

8. Probiotics, prebiotics, synbiotics and HCV

Probiotics are defined as viable microorganisms might be bacteria or yeasts, which display a beneficial effect on the health of the host consumed. Members of the genera *Lactococcus* and *Lactobacillus* are stated as the most common and generally safe [53]. The definition of probiotics by the United Nations and WHO is: *live microorganisms which when directed in adequate amounts converse a health benefit for the host* [54].

Probiotics, which contain the genus *Bacillus*, are supposed to reduce *Staphylococcus aureus* species in the intestines and proliferate their colonisation in the nares. The suggestion that eradication of HCV increases the numbers of *Bacillus* spp. and thus causes a reduction in infection occurrence from bacteria such as *S. aureus*. The development of such a suggestion might be due to the reverse immunosuppression caused by HCV eradication [38].

HCV-positive patients were subjected to a clinical trial to determination of the safety and long-term effect of intake to the probiotic FK-23 which is a heat-treated *Enterococcus faecalis* strain (FK-23). The adjusted amount was 2700 mg of FK-23 each day through oral administration. The alanine aminotransferase (ALT) and aspartate transaminase were determined from blood samples every 3 months. In addition, viral load, urea, total protein, haemoglobin and platelet count were evaluated every 6 months. The results showed a significant decrease in mean ALT levels at 3 months when compared to the initial level and continued up to 36 months. A decrease in AST was identified after 9 months from probiotic therapy when compared to the initial level. The safety of FK-23 was based on the stable levels of measured parameters on biochemical and haematological bases and the lack of side effects. As the Nichinichi Pharmaceutical Co. Ltd. in Japan manufactured functional foods enclosing FK-23, this may contribute to the probiotic industry as an important line in pharmaceutical industries [6].

Probiotic bacteria can diminish hepatocellular carcinoma risk by modifying host gut microbiota [33] to stimulate the growth of beneficial microbes and inhibit HCC-associated dysbiosis, consequently blocking PAMPs, which mediate hepatic inflammation. The antiviral activities from probiotics against HBV and HCV infections ameliorate obesity and the risk of non-alcoholic fatty liver disease NAFLD or non-alcoholic steatohepatitis NASH affect the prevention of HCC pathogenesis. In addition, the antioxidant, anti-proliferative, anti-angiogenic and anti-metastatic effects can inhibit the pathogenesis of HCC. Also, Probiotics have an effect on the upregulation of the expression of tumour suppressor genes and the downregulation of oncogene expression. Additionally, the degradation of dietary phytochemicals by metabolites produced by probiotics may lessen the risk of HCC progress. These several anticancer approaches demonstrate the potential of probiotics as an applied strategy for the risk management and treatment of HCC [55]. Probiotics are known as commensal bacteria including strains of *Lactobacillus* and *Bifidobacterium* species abundant in fermented dairy food. Developing indications directs probiotics use as a therapeutic target for HCC [56, 57].

The reduction of HCC risk was achieved through the probiotic bacteria. There are emerging mechanisms that enrich the host gut microbiome and inhibit dysbiosis-associated endotoxemia. Other preventive activities such as conservation of gut epithelial barrier function and inhibition of gut bacterial translocation and pathogen-associated molecular patterns in the circulation. The ability of probiotic bacteria in the biotransformation of non-nutritional components such as flavonoids and oligosaccharides into effective beneficial metabolites support HCC prevention [55].

Probiotics composed of *Lactobacillus rhamnosus* GG (LGG), viable *Escherichia coli* Nissle 1917 (EcN) and the heat-inactivated VSL#3 with 1:1:1 conformation. VSL#3 comprising *Streptococcus thermophilus*, *Bifidobacterium breve*, *Bifidobacterium longum*, *Bifidobacterium infantis*, *Lactobacillus acidophilus*, *Lactobacillus plantarum*, *Lactobacillus paracasei* and *Lactobacillus delbrueckii* subsp. *Lactobacillus rhamnosus* strain GG (LGG) was extracted from Valio Gefilus capsule and Mutaflor capsules comprising nonpathogenic *Escherichia coli* Nissle 1917 (EcN) bacteria strains. All were used to study the effect of oral feeding of these three individual probiotic preparations on the progression of tumours in the mice HCC model. The results showed that probiotic intake can influence the growth of the gut microbiome, which comprises certain beneficial bacteria such as *Prevotella* and *Oscillibacter* responsible for the production of anti-inflammatory metabolites with the activity of HCC suppression [58].

Prebiotics are known as food ingredients, that have a selective effect on stimulating the growth or activity of beneficial microorganisms such as bacteria and fungi. The synergetic combination between probiotics and prebiotics is called synbiotics. A form of synbiotics, *Lactobacillus paracasei* B21060 and arabinogalactan and fructooligosaccharides (FOSs) (FOSs is a mixture of fermentable dietary fibres) can reduce the hepatic inflammation in diet-induced in non-alcoholic fatty liver disease (NAFLD). The supplementation of seven probiotics consisting of *L. casei*, *L. rhamnosus*, *S. thermophilus*. *Bifidobacterium breve*, *L. acidophilus*, *B. longum* and *L bulgaricus* and FOSs induced the improvement of fasting blood glucose, serum triglycerides in addition to inflammatory cytokines levels in lean and obese patients of NAFLD [59].

On the other side, the use of probiotics should be monitored and in adjusted doses to avoid the side effects on the human body. The usage of some probiotic strains carrying antibiotic resistance genes could lead to the passage of the antibiotic resistance genes to the pathogenic bacteria over the horizontal gene transfer [60]. Probiotic usage should be monitored in consideration of the benefit-to-risk rule and taking in concern the extreme characterisations to both the promise of therapy and the hazard of probiotics [61].

9. Discussion

The human gut microbiome is rich with a diverse microbial community. The identification of species composition through molecular bases allowed the zooming option for precise microbiome balance screening which known to be occur in cases of HCV infection. In *screening studies of gut microbiome between chronic* hepatitis C virus and healthy individuals, most of the studies detected low bacterial diversity in persons with HCV infection. The reduction in the order of Clostridiales and the increase in the *Streptococcus* and *Lactobacillus*. Other factors such as the translocation of molecules from the gut microbiome also affect in variation of liver function and alteration of the pathology of viral hepatitis. The effect of the metabolism of bile acid (BA) in the gut-liver axis through gut microbiota is another mechanism altering patient's overall physiological parameters during disease progress. The overall route of produced secondary microbial metabolites influenced HCV patients' health problems. In addition, screening the microbiome balance during HCV treatment is one of the main factors contributing to the progress of other health problems that emerge from microbial imbalance during a patient's treatment. Based on a number of studies that screened the microbial diversity in HCV patients during treatment, it was noticed that over the long period of treatment, the gut microbiome tends to gain the gut microbial balance. On the other side, the protective immunological function of normal microbiota present in oral and gut microbiome contributes to the overall progress of treatment and thus recurrent infection. The mutual relation between probiotics, prebiotics and synbiotics in contributing to HCV patient's health under treatment and while on medication.

10. Conclusion and future prospective

Despite the effect of the high incidence of HCV infection clearance in last years, there are many studies directed to the long-term effect after treatment. According to the above data, the importance of screening HCV and monitoring the disease progress and consequences on overall health is one of the main targets in reducing the indices in a lower number of cases and thus disease development.

As HCV development causes alterations in the gut microbiome of infected patients even after treatment, the balance of the microbial community could be reached back with the use of probiotics. They are found in food, particularly in fermented dairy products, and could be used up through pharmaceutical preparations. The progress of new probiotic strains targets the most active beneficial microorganisms.

Finally, probiotic bacteria could be used as non-nutritional dietary components. The production of metabolites by beneficial bacteria could enhance the patient's digestive system health, and gain gut microbiome balance thus develop immunity during infection. Also, could contribute to recovery after antiviral treatment. The design of new probiotics based on different therapeutic modes of action could enhance the development of preventive and complementary therapy.

Author details

Naiera M. Helmy
Microbial Biotechnology Department, National Research Centre, Biotechnology Research Institute, Giza, Egypt

*Address all correspondence to: naiera.mohamed@yahoo.com

References

[1] Russo E, Amedei A. The role of the microbiota in the genesis of gastrointestinal cancers. Frontiers in Anti-Infective Drug Discovery. 2018;7:1

[2] Huttenhower C, Gevers D, Knight R, Abubucker S, Badger JH, Chinwalla AT, et al. Structure, function and diversity of the healthy human microbiome. Nature. 2012;**486**(7402):207-214

[3] Li J, Jia H, Cai X, Zhong H, Feng Q, Sunagawa S, et al. An integrated catalog of reference genes in the human gut microbiome. Nature Biotechnology. 2014;**32**(8):834-841

[4] Manos J. The human microbiome in disease and pathology. APMIS. 2022;**130**(12):690-705

[5] Lopetuso LR, Ianiro G, Scaldaferri F, Cammarota G, Gasbarrini A. Gut Virome and inflammatory bowel disease. Inflammatory Bowel Diseases. 2016;**22**(7):1708-1712

[6] Oo KM, Lwin AA, Kyaw YY, Tun WM, Fukada K, Goshima A, et al. Safety and long-term effect of the probiotic FK-23 in patients with hepatitis C virus infection. Bioscience of Microbiota, Food and Health. 2016;**35**(3):123-128

[7] Martinello M, Solomon SS, Terrault NA, Dore GJ. Hepatitis C. Lancet. 2023;**402**(10407):1085-1096

[8] Abdel-Gawad M, Nour M, El-Raey F, Nagdy H, Almansoury Y, El-Kassas M. Gender differences in prevalence of hepatitis C virus infection in Egypt: A systematic review and meta-analysis. Scientific Reports. 2023;**13**(1):2499

[9] Alghamdi AS, Alghamdi H, Alserehi HA, Babatin MA, Alswat KA, Alghamdi M, et al. SASLT guidelines: Update in treatment of hepatitis C virus infection, 2024. Saudi Journal of Gastroenterology. 2024;**30**(Supp 1):S1-S42

[10] Gawlik K, Gallay PA. HCV core protein and virus assembly: What we know without structures. Immunologic Research. 2014;**60**(1):1-10

[11] Martinello M, Naggie S, Rockstroh JK, Matthews GV. Direct-acting antiviral therapy for treatment of acute and recent hepatitis C virus infection: A narrative review. Clinical Infectious Diseases. 2023;**77**(Suppl. 3):S238-s244

[12] Khattab MA, Zakaria Y, Sadek E, El Fatah AS, Fouad M, Khattab M, et al. Abd detection of hepatitis C virus (HCV) RNA in the peripheral blood mononuclear cells of HCV-infected patients following sustained virologic response. Clinical and Experimental Medicine. 2023;**23**(1):131-140

[13] Weersma RK, Zhernakova A, Fu J. Interaction between drugs and the gut microbiome. Gut. 2020;**69**(8):1510-1519

[14] Mallick H, Ma S, Franzosa EA, Vatanen T, Morgan XC, Huttenhower C. Experimental design and quantitative analysis of microbial community multiomics. Genome Biology. 2017;**18**(1):228

[15] Rajagopala SV, Vashee S, Oldfield LM, Suzuki Y, Venter JC, Telenti A, et al. The human microbiome and cancer. Cancer Prevention Research. 2017;**10**(4):226-234

[16] Preveden T, Scarpellini E, Milić N, Luzza F, Abenavoli L. Gut microbiota

changes and chronic hepatitis C virus infection. Expert Review of Gastroenterology & Hepatology. 2017;**11**(9):813-819

[17] Inoue T, Nakayama J, Moriya K, Kawaratani H, Momoda R, Ito K, et al. Gut dysbiosis associated with hepatitis C virus infection. Clinical Infectious Diseases. 2018;**67**(6):869-877

[18] Milosevic I, Russo E, Vujovic A, Barac A, Stevanovic O, Gitto S, et al. Microbiota and viral hepatitis: State of the art of a complex matter. World Journal of Gastroenterology. 2021;**27**(33):5488-5501

[19] Aly AM, Adel A, El-Gendy AO, Essam TM, Aziz RK. Gut microbiome alterations in patients with stage 4 hepatitis C. Gut Pathogens. 2016;**8**(1):42

[20] Iljazovic A, Roy U, Gálvez EJC, Lesker TR, Zhao B, Gronow A, et al. Perturbation of the gut microbiome by *Prevotella* spp. enhances host susceptibility to mucosal inflammation. Mucosal Immunology. 2021;**14**(1):113-124

[21] McBrearty N, Arzumanyan A, Bichenkov E, Merali S, Merali C, Feitelson M. Short chain fatty acids delay the development of hepatocellular carcinoma in HBx transgenic mice. Neoplasia. 2021;**23**(5):529-538

[22] Ullah N, Kakakhel MA, Khan I, Gul Hilal M, Lajia Z, Bai Y, et al. Structural and compositional segregation of the gut microbiota in HCV and liver cirrhotic patients: A clinical pilot study. Microbial Pathogenesis. 2022;**171**:105739

[23] Inoue T, Funatsu Y, Ohnishi M, Isogawa M, Kawashima K, Tanaka M, et al. Bile acid dysmetabolism in the gut-microbiota-liver axis under hepatitis C virus infection. Liver International. 2022;**42**(1):124-134

[24] Jinato T, Anuntakarun S, Satthawiwat N, Chuaypen N, Tangkijvanich P. Distinct alterations of gut microbiota between viral- and non-viral-related hepatocellular carcinoma. Applied Microbiology and Biotechnology. 2024;**108**(1):34

[25] Yang X, Mai H, Zhou J, Li Z, Wang Q, Lan L, et al. Alterations of the gut microbiota associated with the occurrence and progression of viral hepatitis. Frontiers in Cellular and Infection Microbiology. 2023;**13**:1119875

[26] Larrea E, Riezu-Boj JI, Gil-Guerrero L, Casares N, Aldabe R, Sarobe P, et al. Upregulation of indoleamine 2,3-dioxygenase in hepatitis C virus infection. Journal of Virology. 2007;**81**(7):3662-3666

[27] Jenabian MA, Mehraj V, Costiniuk CT, Vyboh K, Kema I, Rollet K, et al. Influence of hepatitis C virus sustained virological response on immunosuppressive tryptophan catabolism in ART-treated HIV/HCV coinfected patients. Journal of Acquired Immune Deficiency Syndromes. 2016;**71**(3):254-262

[28] Feng S, Achoute L, Margolskee RF, Jiang P, Wang H. Lipopolysaccharide-induced inflammatory cytokine expression in taste organoids. Chemical Senses. 2020;**45**(3):187-194

[29] Calder PC. Fatty acids and inflammation: The cutting edge between food and pharma. European Journal of Pharmacology. 2011;**668**(Suppl. 1):S50-S58

[30] Popescu CI, Riva L, Vlaicu O, Farhat R, Rouillé Y, Dubuisson J. Hepatitis C virus life cycle and lipid metabolism. Biology (Basel). 2014;**3**(4):892-921

[31] Bajaj JS, Sterling RK, Betrapally NS, Nixon DE, Fuchs M, Daita K, et al. HCV eradication does not impact gut dysbiosis or systemic inflammation in cirrhotic patients. Alimentary Pharmacology & Therapeutics. 2016;**44**(6):638-643

[32] Ponziani FR, Putignani L, Paroni Sterbini F, Petito V, Picca A, Del Chierico F, et al. Influence of hepatitis C virus eradication with direct-acting antivirals on the gut microbiota in patients with cirrhosis. Alimentary Pharmacology & Therapeutics. 2018;**48**(11-12):1301-1311

[33] Zimmermann M, Zimmermann-Kogadeeva M, Wegmann R, Goodman AL. Separating host and microbiome contributions to drug pharmacokinetics and toxicity. Science. 2019;**363**(6427):8

[34] Pérez-Matute P, Íñiguez M, Villanueva-Millán MJ, Recio-Fernández E, Vázquez AM, Sánchez SC, et al. Short-term effects of direct-acting antiviral agents on inflammation and gut microbiota in hepatitis C-infected patients. European Journal of Internal Medicine. 2019;**67**:47-58

[35] Sultan S, El-Mowafy M, Elgaml A, El-Mesery M, El Shabrawi A, Elegezy M, et al. Alterations of the treatment-naive gut microbiome in newly diagnosed hepatitis C virus infection. ACS Infectious Diseases. 2021;**7**(5):1059-1068

[36] Yilmaz B, Ruckstuhl L, Müllhaupt B, Magenta L, Kuster MH, Clerc O, et al. Pilot sub-study of the effect of hepatitis C cure by glecaprevir/pibrentasvir on the gut microbiome of patients with chronic hepatitis C genotypes 1 to 6 in the mythen study. Pharmaceuticals (Basel). 2021;**14**(9):931

[37] Chuaypen N, Jinato T, Avihingsanon A, Chirapongsathorn S, Cheevadhanarak S, Nookaew I, et al. Improvement of gut diversity and composition after direct-acting antivirals in hepatitis C virus-infected patients with or without human immunodeficiency virus coinfection. The Journal of Infectious Diseases. 2021;**224**(8):1410-1421

[38] Honda T, Ishigami M, Yamamoto K, Takeyama T, Ito T, Ishizu Y, et al. Changes in the gut microbiota after hepatitis C virus eradication. Scientific Reports. 2021;**11**(1):23568

[39] Wellhöner F, Döscher N, Woelfl F, Vital M, Plumeier I, Kahl S, et al. Eradication of chronic HCV infection: Improvement of dysbiosis only in patients without liver cirrhosis. Hepatology. 2021;**74**(1):72-82

[40] Hsu YC, Chen CC, Lee WH, Chang CY, Lee FJ, Tseng CH, et al. Compositions of gut microbiota before and shortly after hepatitis C viral eradication by direct antiviral agents. Scientific Reports. 2022;**12**(1):5481

[41] Ali RO, Quinn GM, Umarova R, Haddad JA, Zhang GY, Townsend EC, et al. Longitudinal multi-omics analyses of the gut-liver axis reveals metabolic dysregulation in hepatitis C infection and cirrhosis. Nature Microbiology. 2023;**8**(1):12-27

[42] Pinchera B, Scotto R, Zappulo E, Buonomo AR, Maraolo AE, Schiano Moriello N, et al. Impact of oral antiviral therapy against HCV on gut microbiota. A prospective study. The New Microbiologica. 2023;**46**(2):196-201

[43] Quinn G, Ali RO, Zhang GY, Hill K, Townsend E, Umarova R, et al. Non-selective dampening of the host immune response after hepatitis C clearance and its association with circulating

chemokine and endotoxin levels. Liver International. 2023;**43**(12):2701-2712

[44] Huang PY, Chen CH, Tsai MJ, Yao CC, Wang HM, Kuo YH, et al. Effects of direct anti-viral agents on the gut microbiota in patients with chronic hepatitis C. Journal of the Formosan Medical Association. 2023;**122**(2):157-163

[45] Wellhöner F, Döscher N, Tergast TL, Vital M, Plumeier I, Kahl S, et al. The impact of proton pump inhibitors on the intestinal microbiota in chronic hepatitis C patients. Scandinavian Journal of Gastroenterology. 2019;**54**(8):1033-1041

[46] Aas JA, Paster BJ, Stokes LN, Olsen I, Dewhirst FE. Defining the normal bacterial flora of the oral cavity. Journal of Clinical Microbiology. 2005;**43**(11):5721-5732

[47] Elghannam MT, Hassanien MH, Ameen YA, Turky EA, Elattar GM, ElRay AA, et al. Oral microbiota and liver diseases. Clinical Nutrition ESPEN. 2023;**54**:68-72

[48] Hernandez BY, Zhu X, Risch HA, Lu L, Ma X, Irwin ML, et al. Oral cyanobacteria and hepatocellular carcinoma. Cancer Epidemiology, Biomarkers & Prevention. 2022;**31**(1):221-229

[49] Gamal-Abdel Naser A, Mohammed WS, ElHefnawi M, Abd Allah M, Elsharkawy A, Zahran FM. The oral microbiome of treated and untreated chronic HCV infection: A preliminary study. Oral Diseases. 2023;**29**(2):843-852

[50] Lee Y-H, Chung SW, Auh Q-S, Hong S-J, Lee Y-A, Jung J, et al. Progress in oral microbiome related to oral and systemic diseases: An update. Diagnostics. 2021;**11**(7):1283

[51] Nagao Y, Sata M, Suzuki H, Kameyama T, Ueno T. Histological improvement of oral lichen planus in patients with chronic hepatitis C treated with interferon. Gastroenterology. 1999;**117**(1):283-284

[52] Di Stasio D, Guida A, Romano A, Petruzzi M, Marrone A, Fiori F, et al. Hepatitis C virus (HCV) infection: Pathogenesis, oral manifestations, and the role of direct-acting antiviral therapy: A narrative review. Journal of Clinical Medicine. 2024;**13**(14):4012

[53] Salminen S, von Wright A, Morelli L, Marteau P, Brassart D, de Vos WM, et al. Demonstration of safety of probiotics—a review. International Journal of Food Microbiology. 1998;**44**(1-2):93-106

[54] Abenavoli L, Luzza F, Mendez-Sanchez N. Probiotics supplementation in the management of hepatocellular carcinoma. Hepatobiliary Surgery and Nutrition. 2019;**8**(6):632-634

[55] Thilakarathna W, Rupasinghe HPV, Ridgway ND. Mechanisms by which probiotic bacteria attenuate the risk of hepatocellular carcinoma. International Journal of Molecular Sciences. 2021;**22**(5):2606

[56] Ponziani FR, Nicoletti A, Gasbarrini A, Pompili M. Diagnostic and therapeutic potential of the gut microbiota in patients with early hepatocellular carcinoma. Therapeutic Advances in Medical Oncology. 2019;**11**:1758835919848184

[57] Milosevic I, Vujovic A, Barac A, Djelic M, Korac M, Radovanovic Spurnic A, et al. Gut-liver axis, gut microbiota, and its modulation in the management of liver diseases: A review of the literature. International Journal of Molecular Sciences. 2019;**20**(2):395

[58] Li J, Sung CY, Lee N, Ni Y, Pihlajamäki J, Panagiotou G, et al. Probiotics modulated gut microbiota suppresses hepatocellular carcinoma growth in mice. Proceedings of the National Academy of Sciences of the United States of America. 2016;**113**(9):E1306-E1315

[59] Wang L, Wan YY. The role of gut microbiota in liver disease development and treatment. Liver Research. 2019;**3**(1):3-18

[60] Imperial IC, Ibana JA. Addressing the antibiotic resistance problem with probiotics: Reducing the risk of its double-edged sword effect. Frontiers in Microbiology. 2016;**7**:1983

[61] Sharp RR, Achkar JP, Brinich MA, Farrell RM. Helping patients make informed choices about probiotics: A need for research. The American Journal of Gastroenterology. 2009;**104**(4):809-813

Chapter 6

Surpassing Viral Suppression: A Breakthrough from Interferon for the Treatment of Hepatitis B

Jiafeng Ge, Haonan Zhao, Pengpeng Xie, Xingshun Qi and Chengwei Tang

Abstract

Hepatitis B virus (HBV) remains a major global public health issue, posing significant threats to human health and quality of life. Its treatment has always been the focus of contemporary medicine. Compared with traditional antiviral drugs, pegylated interferon (Peg-IFN), as an important drug for treating chronic hepatitis B (CHB), is expected to achieve functional cure. In addition, IFN has shown definite efficacy and advantages in inhibiting viral replication, improving liver inflammation, and reducing the risk of liver cirrhosis and hepatocellular carcinoma. However, due to significant side effects and poor compliance, IFN faces many challenges. This chapter systematically analyzes the mechanisms underlying IFN therapy as well as current advances in clinical research regarding IFN for the treatment of CHB.

Keywords: hepatitis B virus, interferon, peg-interferon, treatment, antiviral agents, advances

1. Introduction

Hepatitis B virus (HBV) infection is a major global public health concern. The World Health Organization (WHO) launched a goal of comprehensive HBV elimination in 2016, aiming to reduce new infection rate by 90% and decrease its related mortality rates by 65% by 2030 [1]. Although the global rate of HBV infection has decreased with the use of preventive vaccines, the global burden of HBV remains significant [2]. According to the recent statistics, the global prevalence of HBV infection in 2022 was estimated to be 3.2%, corresponding to 257.5 million individuals living with chronic HBV infection [2]. However, only 36 million individuals had been diagnosed (<14%), and just 6.8 million were receiving treatment. These gaps in diagnosis and treatment remain major barriers to HBV elimination. In addition, HBV prevalence shows significant geographical differences, with higher burden observed in low-income countries or regions, while lower burden was reported in high-income countries or regions [2–4]. Notably, HBV treatment coverage does not appear to correlate with regional economic development, and the management of HBV remains unsatisfactory in high-income countries or regions [5].

HBV can cause either acute or chronic infections. Acute infections may be asymptomatic or have non-specific symptoms, including nausea, fatigue, or jaundice, which are easily overlooked or misattributed to other causes [6]. In addition, individuals with chronic hepatitis B (CHB) are typically asymptomatic for years or even decades and are often identified incidentally through routine health screening, which poses a greater long-term health risk [7]. This asymptomatic nature, coupled with low public awareness and insufficient screening, contributes to the low diagnostic rate of HBV globally. This underdiagnosis not only delays timely antiviral intervention but also increases the risk of disease progression to cirrhosis and hepatocellular carcinoma (HCC).

HBV is a hepatotropic virus characterized by the persistent presence of covalently closed circular DNA (cccDNA) within infected hepatocytes [8]. Therefore, the elimination of cccDNA is crucial for managing CHB [9]. Antiviral therapies for CHB, such as nucleos(t)ide analogs (NAs), which include entecavir (ETV), tenofovir disoproxil fumarate (TDF), and tenofovir alafenamide (TAF), have been shown to significantly delay the progression of liver fibrosis and lower the risk of HCC in CHB patients [10, 11] [12]. Although NAs can suppress HBV replication, they do not directly inhibit the transcriptional activity of cccDNA to achieve the disappearance of HBsAg. Compared to NAs, pegylated interferon (Peg-IFN), as an immunomodulator, can suppress HBV transcription and decrease the expression of HBsAg through epigenetic modification of cccDNA. Multiple guidelines have recommended it as a promising therapy for achieving a functional cure of HBV [13–15]. However, IFN treatment also has some limitations, such as numerous side effects and poor responses in some patients [16].

Therefore, a thorough understanding of the role of IFN for the treatment of HBV is of clinical importance. This chapter aims to summarize the classification of IFN, the mechanism of its treatment for HBV, and the advances in clinical research.

2. Pathogenesis and diagnosis of HBV

2.1 Life cycle of HBV

HBV is an enveloped DNA virus with a genome of about 3.2 kbp, belonging to the *Hepadnaviridae* family [17–20]. HBV exhibits a tropism for hepatocytes and initiates its replication cycle via reverse transcription [21]. Infection begins when the HBsAg within the viral envelope binds in a low-affinity interaction with hepatocyte heparan sulphate proteoglycans (HSPGs) [22], followed by a highly specific binding between the N-terminal preS1 domain of the large surface protein (L-HBsAg) and the sodium taurocholate cotransporting polypeptide (NTCP), which triggers endocytosis of the virion into hepatocytes [23–25]. Upon entering the hepatocytes, the nucleocapsid is released relaxed circular DNA (rcDNA) into the cytoplasm, which is transported to the nucleus and repaired into cccDNA minichromosomes [26–29]. cccDNA serves as the stable transcriptional template for viral RNAs, including pregenomic RNA (pgRNA) and subgenomic mRNAs, through host RNA polymerase II, and persists in hepatocyte nucleus for long [26, 27, 30]. Viral replication occurs within the capsid and the nucleocapsid, where pgRNA is reversely transcribed by the viral polymerase. Approximately, 10% of the pgRNA is reversely transcribed into double-stranded linear DNA (dslDNA), which can integrate into the host genome, thereby contributing to viral persistence and increasing the risk of cirrhosis and HCC. The remaining 90% of pgRNA is reversely transcribed into rcDNA [7, 31, 32]. The rcDNA-containing capsids either recycle to the nucleus to sustain the cccDNA pool or undergo envelopment to form infectious virions for secretion [17, 27, 33].

2.2 Immunological mechanism of HBV

HBV infection is non-cytopathic, indicating that it does not directly kill hepatocytes. Instead, it destroys the infected hepatocytes through host immune response, leading to hepatic inflammation and necrosis [34, 35]. Intermittent and repetitive nature of this process, as well as its related liver injury, may further increase the risk of HCC [7].

The immunological characteristics of CHB infection is the absence of an effective and coordinated adaptive immune response, leading to incomplete viral clearance and persistent infection [21, 34]. A major contributor to this immune dysfunction is the presence of large quantities of subviral particles, which are predominantly composed of HBsAg. These particles inhibit innate immune responses by downregulating the transcription of pro-inflammatory cytokines and interferon-stimulated genes (ISGs) [36–38]. In addition, they also weaken T cell responses, causing T cell "exhaustion" and dysfunction of virus-specific T cells ($CD4^+$ and $CD8^+$ T cells) [39, 40]. In CHB infection, the frequency and function of intrahepatic and peripheral HBV-specific T cells correlate negatively with circulating HBV DNA levels, indicating ongoing immune suppression in the presence of high viral load [41]. Furthermore, the immune dysfunction extends from T cells to multiple other components of the immune system, such as HBsAg-specific B cells, dendritic cells, and NK cells [42]. Apart from the immune mechanisms mentioned above, the inherently immunosuppressive properties of the hepatic microenvironment—while protecting against severe inflammation—also impair HBV-specific T cell function [43]. These processes can lead to chronic inflammation of the liver and subsequently to fibrosis [44].

2.3 Serologic markers and diagnosis of HBV

2.3.1 Serologic markers

The detection of serological markers plays an important role in the diagnosis of HBV. The HBV genome contains four overlapping open reading frames (ORFs), which define the coding capacity of the HBV genome [19, 34]. They can encode seven distinct proteins, including HBsAg (large, medium and small), HBV core antigen (HBcAg), HBV e antigen (HBeAg), HBV polymerase (pol), and the trans-activating transcription factor hepatitis B X protein (HBx) [17]. Currently, the markers that are detectable by commercial serologic tests are HBsAg, HBeAg, anti-HBs, anti-HBc, anti-HBe, and HBV DNA, which are mainly detected through immunoassay methods [45, 46].

HBsAg and anti-HBs: HBsAg is a key structural component of the viral envelope and serves as a major marker of HBV infection [46, 47]. It typically can be detected several weeks after exposure to the HBV [48, 49]. The titer of HBsAg reaches its peak at the height of clinical illness and decreases during the recovery period [50]. The quantitative measurement of HBsAg has been incorporated into the risk scores for predicting HCC as well as evaluating the risk of viral rebound after the discontinuation of NAs [51]. Following the clearance of HBsAg, the emergence of anti-HBs, referred to as HBsAg seroconversion, marks recovery and is associated with viral suppression and favorable prognosis [48]. Anti-HBs seropositivity can also result from effective vaccination or natural resolution of acute HBV [34].

HBeAg and anti-HBe: HBeAg is a soluble dimeric protein secreted by hepatocytes infected with HBV, derived from the processing of the pre-C protein [27, 52]. It can be detected during the acute infection period 6 to 12 weeks after exposure to HBV and is associated with the replication activity and high infectivity of the virus [48, 53]. Seroconversion from HBeAg to anti-HBe positivity is indicative of reduced viral replication and improved hepatic inflammation [53].

Anti-HBc: Total anti-HBc serves as a serological marker for identifying individuals with current or prior HBV infection, typically appearing at early stage of infection [54, 55]. It includes two subtypes: IgM levels rise significantly in acute hepatitis B infection, while IgG levels increase in chronic infections [54]. Total anti-HBc may persist for life, but it may not be detectable in immunocompromised individuals [56, 57]. Serum anti-HBc levels have also been recognized as markers for evaluating the therapeutic efficacy of NAs and Peg-IFN in patients with CHB [58, 59]. Accordingly, the measurement of anti-HBc is typically employed in patients suspected with acute exacerbation of CHB or for determining the need for prophylactic antiviral therapy in patients scheduled to receive immunosuppressive treatment [34, 60].

HBV-DNA: HBV DNA level directly reflects viral replication activity, serves as a diagnostic marker for HBV infection, and can be detected within 2 weeks after primary infection [49, 61]. Quantitative real-time polymerase chain reaction is the most widely used method for HBV DNA detection, owing to its high sensitivity and specificity [62]. Achieving and maintaining undetectable serum HBV DNA levels is a key goal of antiviral therapy [34, 62] Notably, patients who are negative for HBsAg but positive for HBV DNA are referred to as having "occult" HBV infection [63]. Therefore, all CHB patients should have regular monitoring of HBV DNA for the detection of the emergence of viral drug resistance and drug compliance [64].

2.3.2 Diagnosis of HBV

The diagnosis of CHB is primarily based on serological markers, with the persistence of HBsAg for more than 6 months serving as the defining criterion [7, 27].

3. Nature history of HBV

The natural history of HBV can be divided based on virological, serological, clinical manifestations, and histological characteristics and defined by serum transaminases and related biomarkers, providing a critical foundation for defining clinical phenotypes and informing treatment strategies [15]. According to the EASL clinical practice guidelines of HBV, the main stages of CHB have been defined as: (I) HBeAg-positive chronic infection, (II) HBeAg-positive CHB, (III) HBeAg-negative chronic infection, and (IV) HBeAg-negative CHB [12, 14].

The first stage mainly occurs in perinatal period or early childhood period [27], characterized by high HBV DNA levels, positive HBsAg and HBeAg, minimally elevated ALT, and absent or minimal hepatic inflammation or fibrosis [65–67]. However, disease progression is possible, warranting regular monitoring [65]. The second stage is characterized by active HBV infection [68], where patients exhibit hepatic inflammation and elevated ALT levels, and may experience either spontaneous or treatment-induced HBeAg seroconversion [69, 70]. As the immune response intensifies, the risk of cirrhosis and HCC increases [16, 66, 71]. Antiviral treatment at this stage is strongly recommended to reduce liver injury and promote HBeAg seroconversion [16]. Upon seroconversion, patients typically transition into the third stage, which is characterized by normal ALT, low or undetectable HBV DNA, and the presence of anti-HBe antibodies [27, 67]. Patients at this stage constitute the largest group of patients with CHB infection [66], with approximately 0.5–2% of patients achieving spontaneous HBsAg clearance annually [27]. The appearance of anti-HBe antibodies may be a signal of disease remission and may indicate good prognosis. However, some CHB patients may progress to the fourth stage (HBeAg-negative, anti-HBe-positive), typically being older, persistent inflammation, fluctuating HBV DNA and ALT levels, and elevated risk of fibrosis progression [66]. Notably, HBV reactivation occurs in approximately 30–40% of patients within 10 years of HBeAg seroconversion, regardless spontaneous or treatment-induced [16]. Therefore, sustained HBsAg clearance is considered the optimal treatment endpoint for HBeAg-negative patients.

4. Conventional interferon for hepatitis B

As previously discussed, cccDNA is the cornerstone of persistent HBV infection. The virus's ability to sustain itself is also closely linked to its immune evasion mechanisms. Current clinical treatment strategies primarily include NAs and IFNs [13, 34, 72]. NAs can effectively inhibit HBV reverse transcription, thereby suppressing viral replication. However, they have limited ability to directly eliminate cccDNA, resulting in inadequate long-term control over immune evasion [73]. Compared to NAs, IFN can directly inhibit the viral life cycle and restore the host's antiviral immunity. Studies indicated that IFN significantly enhances the clearance rate of HBsAg, which is regarded as a critical marker of reversing HBV immune escape [74, 75]. It demonstrates unique therapeutic advantages of IFN in achieving functional cure.

4.1 Type of conventional interferons

IFNs are a group of cytokines first identified in 1957 [76]. They are produced in response to viral infections or double-stranded RNA and function as an immunomodulator against various viruses [13, 77]. Based on structural differences, receptor types, and biological functions, INFs are mainly classified into three types: Type I (including IFN-α, IFN-β, etc.), Type II (IFN-γ), and Type III (IFN-λ) [5, 72, 78]. IFN-α is the primary drug approved for treating HBV[97], which consists of several subtypes, including IFN-α2a and IFN-α2b, and each potentially exhibiting its distinct activity characteristic [79]. Currently, approximately 23 natural IFN-α subtypes have been identified, and recombinant IFN-α molecules, which are generated by recombining different sequence fragments through DNA recombination technology, have demonstrated enhanced antiviral efficacy [80]. Notably, studies suggest that combining IFN-α or IFN-β with IFN-γ may be more effective than using type I IFN alone [81]. Thus, the efficacy of IFN-γ has not been clearly confirmed [6].

4.2 Structure

Most human IFN-α proteins consist of 189 amino acids (188 in the IFN-α2 subtype), with 23 removed as signal peptides during posttranslational modification [80]. It comprises five α-helical bundles linked by loops, with two disulfide bonds formed by four conserved cysteine residues, and Cys29 - Cys139 bond being critical for biological activity [82–85]. These structural characteristics are critical for the antiviral and immunomodulatory functions.

4.3 Antiviral mechanisms

IFNs exert antiviral effects indirectly by binding to specific cell membrane receptors, rather than targeting viruses directly (**Figure 1**) [86–88]. In HBV treatment, IFN-α stimulates the expression of ISGs to directly inhibit viral replication and simultaneously activates immune responses to enhance host antiviral defense [6]. Specifically, upon binding to the IFN-α/β receptor (IFNAR), IFN-α triggers the JAK-STAT signaling pathway, thereby promoting ISGs expression [89]. These ISGs encode antiviral effectors that interfere with various stages of the HBV life cycle and modulate host immune responses [6, 78]. For example, SAMD4A mediates viral RNA degradation by binding to the SRE site in viral RNA [90], while MX2 reduces cccDNA transcription into RNA [91]. In terms of immune regulation, IFN-α can activate various immune cells, such as macrophages, NK cells, dendritic cells, and T cells, which in turn secrete cytokines to regulate the differentiation and activation of B cells and T cells [92]. Additionally, IFN-α can suppresses cccDNA minichromosome activity *via* inhibiting histone deacetylases, resulting in decreased expression of HBsAg and HBeAg, thereby limiting cccDNA

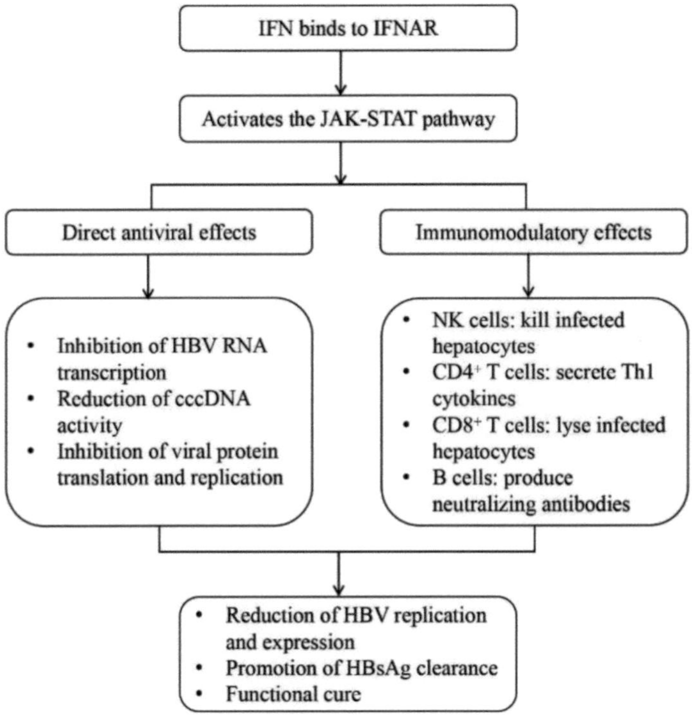

Figure 1.
Mechanism of IFN in the treatment of HBV. IFN, interferon; IFNAR, interferon-α/β receptor; JAK-STAT, Janus kinase-signal transducer and activator of transcription; HBV, hepatitis B virus; RNA, ribonucleic acid; DNA, deoxyribonucleic acid; NK, natural killer; HBsAg, hepatitis B surface antigen.

replenishment [93, 94]. Therefore, IFN therapy is the most effective during the host's immune clearance phase [95].

4.4 Clinical research

Efficacy and limitations of IFN-α have been systematically evaluated since it was approved for CHB in the 1980s. Müller et al. demonstrated a significantly higher response rate in the treatment group with IFN-α-2b than nontreatment group [96]. Meta-analyses also showed superior virological and histological outcomes with IFN [97, 98]. Extending treatment to 32 weeks can effectively improve HBeAg seroconversion [99]. Long-term studies have confirmed that IFN therapy improves outcomes and reduces the risk of cirrhosis and HCC over 15 years [100]. Notably, the effect of conventional IFN not only varies with dose and treatment duration but also is affected by patient characteristics, such as gender, ALT level, and HBV DNA level [98, 101]. However, IFN therapy has some limitations, including significant side effects, such as flu-like symptoms and hematological abnormalities, frequent injections, and high costs [99, 101], which limit its use.

5. Pegylated interferon

The clinical application of conventional IFNs is limited by their short half-life and toxicity. To address these issues, structural modifications have been implemented through pegylation, resulting in improved pharmacokinetics and therapeutic effect (**Table 1**).

5.1 Structure and classification

Peg-IFNs are engineered by covalently conjugating polyethylene glycol (PEG) to IFN molecules. The antiviral efficacy and pharmacokinetics of Peg-IFNs are primarily

Comparison dimension	Conventional IFN	Peg-IFN
Molecular structure	Identical to natural human interferon	Conjugated with PEG molecules
Half-life	Short (approx. 4–6 hours)	Long (approx. 40–80 hours, varies by PEG molecular weight)
Administration frequency	Subcutaneous injection three times per week	Subcutaneous injection once weekly
Plasma concentration stability	High fluctuations, prone to "peak-valley effect"	Steady concentration, maintains therapeutic levels over extended periods
Bioavailability	Lower efficiency, partial clearance before activation	Higher efficiency, PEG modification reduces renal excretion and immune clearance
Therapeutic efficacy	Slightly inferior antiviral and immunomodulatory effects due to concentration fluctuations	Enhanced antiviral and immunomodulatory effects under sustained therapeutic levels
Side effects	Fever, fatigue, flu-like symptoms	Fever, fatigue, flu-like symptoms

IFN, interferon; Peg-IFN, pegylated-interferon; PEG, polyethylene glycol.

Table 1.
Conventional interferon vs. Pegylated interferon.

determined by the molecular weight, conjugation sites, and molecular configuration of the PEG, which prolongs serum half-life without significantly altering the secondary or tertiary structure of the native IFNs [102, 103]. There are two main subtypes: (1) Peg-IFN α-2a: 40 kDa branched PEG conjugated to IFN α-2a *via* lysine residues (dosed by 180 μg/week), suitable for CHB with prolonged half-life (80 hours). (2) Peg-IFN α-2b: 12 kDa linear PEG conjugated to IFN α-2b via His [34] residue or lysine, dosed by weight (1.5 μg/kg/week), with a 40-hour half-life and retained bioactivity, which is suitable for situations where quick results are needed [102–104].

5.2 Clinical research of monotherapy

In HBeAg-positive patients with chronic hepatitis B, Peg-IFNα-2a was more effective than conventional IFNα-2a [104]. Li et al. reported that HBeAg-negative patients switching from NAs to 48 weeks of Peg-IFNα-2a had significantly reduced virological relapse rates and increased HBsAg loss, compared to those discontinuing NAs [105]. An RCT also showed that 68 weeks of Peg-IFNα-2b monotherapy resulted in a high HBsAg loss rate among HBsAg carriers [106] Although their differences in molecular structure and pharmacokinetics, Peg-IFN α-2a and α-2b exhibited comparable efficacy [107]. Notably, HBV genotype influences clinical effect: genotype A shows the best response in HBeAg-positive patients, genotypes B and C have similar performance in Asian patients, and genotype D yields the worst response [107].

5.3 Clinical research of combination with NAs therapy

Peg-IFN is often combined with first-line NAs, such as ETV and TDF, for the management of CHB. This combination therapy capitalizes Peg-IFN's immunomodulatory effects and NAs' antiviral effects to suppress viral replication and reduce the cccDNA pool in hepatocytes more effectively [12]. But this approach is not recommended for all patients. It should be selected based on disease activity, HBV DNA, HBsAg, and HBeAg status. Notably, *de novo* combination therapy is not recommended [12]. Multiple studies have found that the available effective combination treatment methods were mainly based on long-term NAs treatment accompanied by additional Peg-IFN-α therapy [108, 109]. Lim et al. found that HBeAg-negative patients achieved greater HBsAg decline and clearance with combination therapy as compared to HBeAg-positive patients [110]. Switching directly from NAs to Peg-IFN monotherapy may increase the risk of virologic relapse. Therefore, add-on Peg-IFN therapy is preferred. Additionally, in HBeAg-negative CHB patients who had been on long-term NAs treatment and had complete viral suppression for at least 2–3 years, the HBsAg levels significantly decreased in patients treated with Peg-IFN α add-on therapy [111]. Another study showed that regardless of HBeAg status, patients treated with a limited course of Peg-IFN plus TDF had a higher HBsAg loss rate compared to those receiving monotherapy [112]. Beyond NAs-based combinations, emerging combination strategies are under active clinical investigation. For example, the combination of Peg-IFN with novel direct-acting antiviral drugs (DAAs) or novel immunomodulators, including T-cell receptor agonists, checkpoint inhibitors, therapeutic vaccines, and monoclonal antibodies, is also considered a promising treatment approach [109]. Overall, the combination treatment has gradually become an important treatment option for CHB in clinical practice. With the continuous development of immunotherapy and new antiviral drugs, there may be more combined treatment options available in the future to provide better treatment choices for hepatitis B patients.

5.4 Clinical studies of combination with emerging antiviral agents

Combination of Peg-IFN with emerging antiviral agents, such as cccDNA inhibitors and immune checkpoint inhibitors, has become a major focus in the pursuit of functional cure for HBV. A preclinical study demonstrated that cucurbitacin I combined with PEG-IFNα effectively reduced intrahepatic cccDNA levels [113]. The combination of PEG-IFN and small interfering RNA (siRNA) shows even more promise. Both HBsAg seroclearance and anti-HBs seroconversion rates were significantly higher in patients receiving VIR-2218 combined with PEG-IFN for 44 weeks than monotherapy [114, 115]. The synergistic effects between PEG-IFN and capsid assembly modulators (CAMs) have also been validated. For instance, a triple therapy regimen consisting of RO7049389, PEG-IFN, and NAs significantly reduced HBsAg, HBeAg, and HBcrAg levels in patients, outperforming mono- or dual-agent regimens [114]. Notably, PEG-IFN combined with immune checkpoint inhibitors enhances T cell activation, promotes HBsAg decline, and improves immune-mediated viral clearance, offering a promising direction for future combination strategies [114, 115].

5.5 Limitations

Although the combination of Peg-IFN with other antiviral agents improve seroconversion rates, it is associated with a higher incidence of adverse events (AEs) compared to monotherapy [116, 117]. Common AEs of Peg-IFN treatment include influenza-like syndrome and leukopeni, which are mostly mild to moderate and can recover after drug withdrawal [118]. Additionally, due to the injection administration method, patient compliance is relatively poor.

6. Conclusion

IFN is important in CHB treatment with dual effects of immune modulation and antiviral activity. The shift from conventional IFN to Peg-IFN has advanced HBV treatment toward functional cure. Emerging combination strategies, such as Peg-IFN with cccDNA inhibitors or immune checkpoint inhibitors, show significant potential in overcoming immune tolerance and targeting persistent viral reservoirs. However, several real-world barriers must be addressed, including variable patient responses and treatment-related adverse effects. Key strategies to overcome these challenges include improved adherence through patient education, proactive management of side effects, and incorporation of IFN-based regimens into national programs in resource-limited settings to ensure equitable implementation. In addition, we should conduct head-to-head randomized controlled trials stratified by HBV genotype and strengthen long-term follow-up outcomes on functional cure.

Author details

Jiafeng Ge[1,2†], Haonan Zhao[1,2†], Pengpeng Xie[1,2†], Xingshun Qi[1,2*]
and Chengwei Tang[3*]

1 Department of Gastroenterology, General Hospital of Northern Theater Command (Teaching Hospital of Shenyang Pharmaceutical University), Shenyang, China

2 Department of Clinical Pharmacy, Shenyang Pharmaceutical University, Shenyang, China

3 Department of Gastroenterology, West China Hospital, Sichuan University, Chengdu, China

*Address all correspondence to: xingshunqi@126.com and shcqcdmed@163.com

†Co-first authors

References

[1] World Health Organization.? Global health sector strategy on viral hepatitis 2016-2021. Available from: https://www.who.int/publications/i/item/WHO-HIV-2016.06

[2] Polaris Observatory Collaborators. Global prevalence, cascade of care, and prophylaxis coverage of hepatitis B in 2022: A modelling study. The Lancet Gastroenterology & Hepatology. 2023;**8**(10):879-907

[3] Cui F, Blach S, Manzengo Mingiedi C, et al. Global reporting of progress towards elimination of hepatitis B and hepatitis C. The Lancet Gastroenterology & Hepatology. 2023;**8**(4):332-342

[4] Vo-Quang E, Lemoine M. Global elimination of HBV: Is it really achievable? Journal of Viral Hepatitis. 2024;**31**(Suppl. 2):4-12

[5] Hsu YC, Huang DQ, Nguyen MH. Global burden of hepatitis B virus: Current status, missed opportunities and a call for action. Nature Reviews. Gastroenterology & Hepatology. 2023;**20**(8):524-537

[6] Hillaire MLB, Lawrence P, Lagrange B. IFN-γ: A crucial player in the fight against HBV infection? Immune Network. 2023;**23**(4):e30

[7] Tang LSY, Covert E, Wilson E, Kottilil S. Chronic hepatitis B infection: A review. JAMA. 2018;**319**(17):1802-1813

[8] Tsukuda S, Watashi K. Hepatitis B virus biology and life cycle. Antiviral Research. 2020;**182**:104925

[9] Wang L, Zhu Q, Zhang JD, et al. Discovery of a first-in-class orally available HBV cccDNA inhibitor. Journal of Hepatology. 2023;**78**(4):742-753

[10] Calvaruso V, Craxì A. Regression of fibrosis after HBV antiviral therapy. Is cirrhosis reversible? Liver International. 2014;**34**(Suppl. 1):85-90

[11] Huang DQ, Tran A, Yeh ML, et al. Antiviral therapy substantially reduces HCC risk in patients with chronic hepatitis B infection in the indeterminate phase. Hepatology. 2023;**78**(5):1558-1568

[12] European Association for the Study of the Liver. 2017 clinical practice guidelines on the management of hepatitis B virus infection. Journal of Hepatology. 2017;**67**(2):370-398

[13] Ye J, Chen J. Interferon and hepatitis B: Current and future perspectives. Frontiers in Immunology. 2021;**12**:733364

[14] European Association for the Study of the Liver. EASL clinical practice guidelines on the management of hepatitis B virus infection. Journal of Hepatology. 2025;**83**(2):502-583

[15] WHO. Guidelines for the Prevention, Diagnosis, Care and Treatment for People with Chronic Hepatitis B Infection. Geneva: World Health Organization; 2024. Licence: CC BY-NC-SA 3.0 IGO

[16] Chen T-CTJ-HKD-S. Peginterferon α in the treatment of chronic hepatitis B. Expert Opinion on Biological Therapy. 2014;**14**:995-1006

[17] Tu T, Budzinska MA, Shackel NA, Urban S. HBV DNA integration: Molecular mechanisms and clinical implications. Viruses. 2017;**9**(4):75

[18] Nassal M. HBV cccDNA: Viral persistence reservoir and key obstacle for a cure of chronic hepatitis B. Gut. 2015;**64**(12):1972-1984

[19] Hatzakis A, Magiorkinis E, Haida C. HBV virological assessment. Journal of Hepatology. 2006;**44**:S71-SS6

[20] Seitz S, Urban S, Antoni C, Böttcher B. Cryo-electron microscopy of hepatitis B virions reveals variability in envelope capsid interactions. The EMBO Journal. 2007;**26**(18):4160-4167

[21] Lim SG, Baumert TF, Boni C, et al. The scientific basis of combination therapy for chronic hepatitis B functional cure. Nature Reviews. Gastroenterology & Hepatology. 2023;**20**(4):238-253

[22] Sureau C, Salisse J. A conformational heparan sulfate binding site essential to infectivity overlaps with the conserved hepatitis B virus a-determinant. Hepatology. 2013;**57**(3):985-994

[23] Yan H, Zhong G, Xu G, et al. Sodium taurocholate cotransporting polypeptide is a functional receptor for human hepatitis B and D virus. eLife. 2012;**1**:e00049

[24] Schulze A, Gripon P, Urban S. Hepatitis B virus infection initiates with a large surface protein-dependent binding to heparan sulfate proteoglycans. Hepatology. 2007;**46**(6):1759-1768

[25] Blondot ML, Bruss V, Kann M. Intracellular transport and egress of hepatitis B virus. Journal of Hepatology. 2016;**64**(Suppl. 1):S49-s59

[26] Martinez MG, Boyd A, Combe E, Testoni B, Zoulim F. Covalently closed circular DNA: The ultimate therapeutic target for curing HBV infections. Journal of Hepatology. 2021;**75**(3):706-717

[27] HKG DM. Hepatitis B virus: Advances in prevention, diagnosis, and therapy. Clinical Microbiology Reviews. 2020;**33**:e00046-e00019

[28] Schreiner S, Nassal M. A role for the host DNA damage response in hepatitis B virus cccDNA formation-and beyond? Viruses. 2017;**9**(5):125

[29] Newbold JE, Xin H, Tencza M, et al. The covalently closed duplex form of the hepadnavirus genome exists in situ as a heterogeneous population of viral minichromosomes. Journal of Virology. 1995;**69**(6):3350-3357

[30] Tuttleman JS, Pourcel C, Summers J. Formation of the pool of covalently closed circular viral DNA in hepadnavirus-infected cells. Cell. 1986;**47**(3):451-460

[31] Zlotnick A, Venkatakrishnan B, Tan Z, Lewellyn E, Turner W, Francis S. Core protein: A pleiotropic keystone in the HBV lifecycle. Antiviral Research. 2015;**121**:82-93

[32] Tu T, McQuaid TJ, Jacobson IM. HBV-induced carcinogenesis: Mechanisms, correlation with viral suppression, and implications for treatment. Liver International. 2025;**45**(1):e16202

[33] Bock CT, Schwinn S, Locarnini S, et al. Structural organization of the hepatitis B virus minichromosome. Journal of Molecular Biology. 2001;**307**(1):183-196

[34] Yuen MF, Chen DS, Dusheiko GM, et al. Hepatitis B virus infection. Nature Reviews. Disease Primers. 2018;**4**:18035

[35] Baumert TF, Thimme R, von Weizsäcker F. Pathogenesis of hepatitis B virus infection. World Journal of Gastroenterology. 2007;**13**(1):82-90

[36] Shi B, Ren G, Hu Y, Wang S, Zhang Z, Yuan Z. HBsAg inhibits IFN-α production in plasmacytoid dendritic cells through TNF-α and IL-10 induction in monocytes. PLoS One. 2012;7(9):e44900

[37] Jiang M, Broering R, Trippler M, et al. Toll-like receptor-mediated immune responses are attenuated in the presence of high levels of hepatitis B virus surface antigen. Journal of Viral Hepatitis. 2014;**21**(12):860-872

[38] Xu Y, Hu Y, Shi B, et al. HBsAg inhibits TLR9-mediated activation and IFN-alpha production in plasmacytoid dendritic cells. Molecular Immunology. 2009;**46**(13):2640-2646

[39] Chen CF, Feng X, Liao HY, et al. Regulation of T cell proliferation by JMJD6 and PDGF-BB during chronic hepatitis B infection. Scientific Reports. 2014;**4**:6359

[40] Ye B, Liu X, Li X, Kong H, Tian L, Chen Y. T-cell exhaustion in chronic hepatitis B infection: Current knowledge and clinical significance. Cell Death & Disease. 2015;**6**(3):e1694

[41] Webster GJ, Reignat S, Brown D, et al. Longitudinal analysis of CD8+ T cells specific for structural and nonstructural hepatitis B virus proteins in patients with chronic hepatitis B: Implications for immunotherapy. Journal of Virology. 2004;**78**(11):5707-5719

[42] Boeijen LL, Hoogeveen RC, Boonstra A, Lauer GM. Hepatitis B virus infection and the immune response: The big questions. Best Practice & Research. Clinical Gastroenterology. 2017;**31**(3):265-272

[43] Fisicaro P, Barili V, Rossi M, et al. Pathogenetic mechanisms of T cell dysfunction in chronic HBV infection and related therapeutic approaches. Frontiers in Immunology. 2020;**11**:849

[44] Neshat SY, Quiroz VM, Wang Y, Tamayo S, Doloff JC. Liver disease: Induction, progression, immunological mechanisms, and therapeutic interventions. International Journal of Molecular Sciences. 2021;**22**(13):6777

[45] Wang Y, Liu Y, Liao H, et al. Serum HBV DNA plus RNA reflecting cccDNA level before and during NAs treatment in HBeAg positive CHB patients. International Journal of Medical Sciences. 2022;**19**(5):858-866

[46] Chu CM, Liaw YF. Hepatitis B surface antigen seroclearance during chronic HBV infection. Antiviral Therapy. 2010;**15**(2):133-143

[47] Lee JM, Ahn SH. Quantification of HBsAg: Basic virology for clinical practice. World Journal of Gastroenterology. 2011;**17**(3):283-289

[48] Keating GM, Noble S. Recombinant hepatitis B vaccine (Engerix-B): A review of its immunogenicity and protective efficacy against hepatitis B. Drugs. 2003;**63**(10):1021-1051

[49] Zamor PJ, Lane AM. Interpretation of HBV serologies. Clinics in Liver Disease. 2021;**25**(4):689-709

[50] Garrison MW, Baker DE. Therapeutic advances in the prevention of hepatitis B: Yeast-derived recombinant hepatitis B vaccines. DICP. 1991;**25**(6):617-627

[51] Cornberg M, Wong VW, Locarnini S, Brunetto M, Janssen HLA, Chan HL. The role of quantitative hepatitis B surface antigen revisited. Journal of Hepatology. 2017;**66**(2):398-411

[52] Lee WM. Hepatitis B virus infection. The New England Journal of Medicine. 1997;**337**(24):1733-1745

[53] Bonino F, Brunetto MR. Chronic hepatitis B e antigen (HBeAg) negative, anti-HBe positive hepatitis B: An overview. Journal of Hepatology. 2003;**39**(Suppl. 1):S160-S163

[54] Yano Y, Sato I, Imanishi T, et al. Clinical significance and remaining issues of anti-HBc antibody and HBV core-related antigen. Diagnostics (Basel). 2024;**14**(7):728

[55] Schmidt M, Nübling CM, Scheiblauer H, et al. Anti-HBc screening of blood donors: A comparison of nine anti-HBc tests. Vox Sanguinis. 2006;**91**(3):237-243

[56] Holtkamp C, Fiedler M, Dittmer U, Anastasiou OE. The course of anti-HBc antibodies over time in immunocompromised hosts. Vaccines (Basel). 2022;**10**(2):137

[57] Anastasiou OE, Widera M, Verheyen J, et al. Clinical course and core variability in HBV infected patients without detectable anti-HBc antibodies. Journal of Clinical Virology. 2017;**93**:46-52

[58] Fan R, Sun J, Yuan Q, et al. Baseline quantitative hepatitis B core antibody titre alone strongly predicts HBeAg seroconversion across chronic hepatitis B patients treated with peginterferon or nucleos(t)ide analogues. Gut. 2016;**65**(2):313-320

[59] Fang YQ, Xu XY, Hou FQ, Jia W. A baseline model including quantitative anti-HBc to predict response of peginterferon in HBeAg-positive chronic hepatitis B patients. Antiviral Therapy. 2021;**26**(6-8):126-133

[60] Lalazar G, Rund D, Shouval D. Screening, prevention and treatment of viral hepatitis B reactivation in patients with haematological malignancies. British Journal of Haematology. 2007;**136**(5):699-712

[61] Hoofnagle JH, Di Bisceglie AM. Serologic diagnosis of acute and chronic viral hepatitis. Seminars in Liver Disease. 1991;**11**(2):73-83

[62] Coffin CS, Zhou K, Terrault NA. New and old biomarkers for diagnosis and management of chronic hepatitis B virus infection. Gastroenterology. 2019;**156**(2):355-68.e3

[63] de Almeida NAA, de Paula VS. Occult hepatitis B virus (HBV) infection and challenges for hepatitis elimination: A literature review. Journal of Applied Microbiology. 2022;**132**(3):1616-1635

[64] Hongthanakorn C, Chotiyaputta W, Oberhelman K, et al. Virological breakthrough and resistance in patients with chronic hepatitis B receiving nucleos(t)ide analogues in clinical practice. Hepatology. 2011;**53**(6):1854-1863

[65] Mason WS, Gill US, Litwin S, et al. HBV DNA integration and clonal hepatocyte expansion in chronic hepatitis B patients considered immune tolerant. Gastroenterology. 2016;**151**(5):986-98.e4

[66] Shi YH, Shi CH. Molecular characteristics and stages of chronic hepatitis B virus infection. World Journal of Gastroenterology. 2009;**15**(25):3099-3105

[67] Zhang YY, Hu KQ. Rethinking the pathogenesis of hepatitis B virus (HBV) infection. Journal of Medical Virology. 2015;**87**(12):1989-1999

[68] Lin CL, Kao JH. Natural history of acute and chronic hepatitis B: The role of HBV genotypes and mutants.

Best Practice & Research. Clinical Gastroenterology. 2017;**31**(3):249-255

[69] Brunetto MR, Giarin MM, Oliveri F, et al. Wild-type and e antigen-minus hepatitis B viruses and course of chronic hepatitis. Proceedings of the National Academy of Sciences of the United States of America. 1991;**88**(10):4186-4190

[70] Wang HY, Chien MH, Huang HP, et al. Distinct hepatitis B virus dynamics in the immunotolerant and early immunoclearance phases. Journal of Virology. 2010;**84**(7):3454-3463

[71] Furusyo N, Nakashima H, Kashiwagi K, et al. Clinical outcomes of hepatitis B virus (HBV) genotypes B and C in Japanese patients with chronic HBV infection. The American Journal of Tropical Medicine and Hygiene. 2002;**67**(2):151-157

[72] Li Q, Sun B, Zhuo Y, et al. Interferon and interferon-stimulated genes in HBV treatment. Frontiers in Immunology. 2022;**13**:1034968

[73] Levrero M, Subic M, Villeret F, Zoulim F. Perspectives and limitations for nucleo(t)side analogs in future HBV therapies. Current Opinion in Virology. 2018;**30**:80-89

[74] Tan G, Song H, Xu F, Cheng G. When hepatitis B virus meets interferons. Frontiers in Microbiology. 2018;**9**:1611

[75] Lei Z, Wang L, Gao H, et al. Mechanisms underlying the compromised clinical efficacy of interferon in clearing HBV. Virology Journal. 2024;**21**(1):314

[76] Isaacs A, Lindenmann J. Pillars article: Virus interference. I. The interferon. Proc R Soc Lond B biol Sci. 1957. 147: 258-267. Journal of Immunology. 2015;**195**(5):1911-1920

[77] Pestka S, Krause CD, Walter MR. Interferons, interferon-like cytokines, and their receptors. Immunological Reviews. 2004;**202**:8-32

[78] Hoffmann HH, Schneider WM, Rice CM. Interferons and viruses: An evolutionary arms race of molecular interactions. Trends in Immunology. 2015;**36**(3):124-138

[79] Ortaldo JR, Herberman RB, Harvey C, et al. A species of human alpha interferon that lacks the ability to boost human natural killer activity. Proceedings of the National Academy of Sciences of the United States of America. 1984;**81**(15):4926-4929

[80] El-Baky NA, Redwan EM. Therapeutic alpha-interferons protein: Structure, production, and biosimilar. Preparative Biochemistry & Biotechnology. 2015;**45**(2):109-127

[81] Carreno V, Mora I. Combination of recombinant interferons alpha and gamma in treatment of chronic hepatitis B. Lancet. 1987;**2**(8567):1086

[82] Wetzel R. Assignment of the disulphide bonds of leukocyte interferon. Nature. 1981;**289**(5798):606-607

[83] Mitsui Y, Senda T, Shimazu T, Matsuda S, Utsumi J. Structural, functional and evolutionary implications of the three-dimensional crystal structure of murine interferon-beta. Pharmacology & Therapeutics. 1993;**58**(1):93-132

[84] Camble R, Petter NN, Trueman P, et al. Functionally important conserved amino-acids in interferon-alpha 2 identified with analogues produced from synthetic genes. Biochemical and Biophysical Research Communications. 1986;**134**(3):1404-1411

[85] Runkel L, Pfeffer L, Lewerenz M, et al. Differences in activity between alpha and beta type I interferons explored by mutational analysis. The Journal of Biological Chemistry. 1998;**273**(14):8003-8008

[86] Brassard DL, Grace MJ, Bordens RW. Interferon-alpha as an immunotherapeutic protein. Journal of Leukocyte Biology. 2002;**71**(4):565-581

[87] Pfeffer LM, Dinarello CA, Herberman RB, et al. Biological properties of recombinant alpha-interferons: 40th anniversary of the discovery of interferons. Cancer Research. 1998;**58**(12):2489-2499

[88] Stark GR, Kerr IM, Williams BR, Silverman RH, Schreiber RD. How cells respond to interferons. Annual Review of Biochemistry. 1998;**67**:227-264

[89] Yuliantie E, Dai X, Yang D, Crack PJ, Wang MW. High-throughput screening for small molecule inhibitors of the type-I interferon signaling pathway. Acta Pharmaceutica Sinica B. 2018;**8**(6):889-899

[90] Wang Y, Fan X, Song Y, et al. SAMD4 family members suppress human hepatitis B virus by directly binding to the Smaug recognition region of viral RNA. Cellular & Molecular Immunology. 2021;**18**(4):1032-1044

[91] Wang YX, Niklasch M, Liu T, et al. Interferon-inducible MX2 is a host restriction factor of hepatitis B virus replication. Journal of Hepatology. 2020;**72**(5):865-876

[92] Thimme R, Dandri M. Dissecting the divergent effects of interferon-alpha on immune cells: Time to rethink combination therapy in chronic hepatitis B? Journal of Hepatology. 2013;**58**(2):205-209

[93] Belloni L, Allweiss L, Guerrieri F, et al. IFN-α inhibits HBV transcription and replication in cell culture and in humanized mice by targeting the epigenetic regulation of the nuclear cccDNA minichromosome. The Journal of Clinical Investigation. 2012;**122**(2):529-537

[94] Yuan Y, Yuan H, Yang G, et al. IFN-α confers epigenetic regulation of HBV cccDNA minichromosome by modulating GCN5-mediated succinylation of histone H3K79 to clear HBV cccDNA. Clinical Epigenetics. 2020;**12**(1):135

[95] Wong GL, Chan HL. Predictors of treatment response in chronic hepatitis B. Drugs. 2009;**69**(16):2167-2177

[96] Müller R, Baumgarten R, Markus R, et al. Low dose alpha interferon treatment in chronic hepatitis B virus infection. Gut. 1993;**34**(Suppl. 2):S97-S98

[97] Sun X, Qin W, Zhou R, Wang L, Li Y, Zhao L. Effect of conventional interferon-alpha in patients with HBeAg-positive chronic hepatitis B: A systematic review and meta-analysis. Journal of Evidence-Based Medicine. 2010;**3**(4):220-225

[98] Wong DK, Cheung AM, O'Rourke K, Naylor CD, Detsky AS, Heathcote J. Effect of alpha-interferon treatment in patients with hepatitis B e antigen-positive chronic hepatitis B. A meta-analysis. Annals of Internal Medicine. 1993;**119**(4):312-323

[99] Janssen HL, Gerken G, Carreño V, et al. Interferon alfa for chronic hepatitis B infection: Increased efficacy of prolonged treatment. The European concerted action on viral hepatitis (EUROHEP). Hepatology. 1999;**30**(1):238-243

[100] Lin S-M, Yu M-L, Lee C-M, et al. Interferon therapy in HBeAg positive

chronic hepatitis reduces progression to cirrhosis and hepatocellular carcinoma. Journal of Hepatology. 2007;**46**(1):45-52

[101] Perrillo RP. Interferon therapy for chronic type B hepatitis: The promise comes of age. Gastroenterology. 1989;**96**(2 Pt 1):532-535

[102] Grace M, Youngster S, Gitlin G, et al. Structural and biologic characterization of pegylated recombinant IFN-alpha2b. Journal of Interferon & Cytokine Research. 2001;**21**(12):1103-1115

[103] Herrington-Symes A, Choi JW, Brocchini S. Interferon dimers: IFN-PEG-IFN. Journal of Drug Targeting. 2017;**25**(9-10):881-890

[104] Cooksley WG, Piratvisuth T, Lee SD, et al. Peginterferon alpha-2a (40 kDa): An advance in the treatment of hepatitis B e antigen-positive chronic hepatitis B. Journal of Viral Hepatitis. 2003;**10**(4):298-305

[105] Li F, Qu L, Liu Y, et al. PegIFN alpha-2a reduces relapse in HBeAg-negative patients after nucleo(s)tide analogue cessation: A randomized-controlled trial. Journal of Hepatology. 2025;**82**(2):211-221

[106] Ning H, Li K, Peng Z, Jin H, Zhao H, Shang J. The efficacy and safety of pegylated interferon α-2b-based immunotherapy for inactive hepatitis B surface antigen carriers. European Journal of Gastroenterology & Hepatology. 2023;**35**(10):1216-1223

[107] Tseng TC, Kao JH, Chen DS. Peginterferon α in the treatment of chronic hepatitis B. Expert Opinion on Biological Therapy. 2014;**14**(7):995-1006

[108] Ghany MG, Buti M, Lampertico P, Lee HM. Guidance on treatment endpoints and study design for clinical trials aiming to achieve cure in chronic hepatitis B and D: Report from the 2022 AASLD-EASL HBV-HDV treatment endpoints conference. Hepatology. 2023;**78**(5):1654-1673

[109] Chang ML, Liaw YF. Emerging therapies for chronic hepatitis B and the potential for a functional cure. Drugs. 2023;**83**(5):367-388

[110] Lim SG, Yang WL, Ngu JH, et al. Switching to or add-on peginterferon in patients on nucleos(t)ide analogues for chronic hepatitis B: The SWAP RCT. Clinical Gastroenterology and Hepatology. 2022;**20**(2):e228-ee50

[111] Vecchi A, Rossi M, Tiezzi C, et al. HBcrAg values may predict virological and immunological responses to pegIFN-α in NUC-suppressed HBeAg-negative chronic hepatitis B. Gut. 2024;**73**(10):1737-1748

[112] Ahn SH, Marcellin P, Ma X, et al. Hepatitis B surface antigen loss with tenofovir disoproxil fumarate plus peginterferon Alfa-2a: Week 120 analysis. Digestive Diseases and Sciences. 2018;**63**(12):3487-3497

[113] Zhao L, Yuan H, Wang Y, et al. p-STAT3-elevated E3 ubiquitin ligase DTX4 confers the stability of HBV cccDNA by ubiquitinating APOBEC3B in liver. Theranostics. 2024;**14**(15):6036-6052

[114] Zhao Q, Liu H, Tang L, et al. Mechanism of interferon alpha therapy for chronic hepatitis B and potential approaches to improve its therapeutic efficacy. Antiviral Research. 2024;**221**:105782

[115] Korkmaz P, Asan A, Karakeçili F, Tekin S, Demirtürk N. New treatment options in chronic hepatitis B: How close

are we to cure? Infectious Diseases and Clinical Microbiology. 2023;**5**(4):267-280

[116] Farag MS, van Campenhout MJH, Sonneveld MJ, et al. Addition of PEG-interferon to long-term nucleos(t)ide analogue therapy enhances HBsAg decline and clearance in HBeAg-negative chronic hepatitis B. Journal of Viral Hepatitis. 2024;**31**(4):197-207

[117] Bourlière M, Rabiega P, Ganne-Carrie N, et al. Effect on HBs antigen clearance of addition of pegylated interferon alfa-2a to nucleos(t)ide analogue therapy versus nucleos(t)ide analogue therapy alone in patients with HBe antigen-negative chronic hepatitis B and sustained undetectable plasma hepatitis B virus DNA: A randomised, controlled, open-label trial. The Lancet Gastroenterology & Hepatology. 2017;**2**(3):177-188

[118] Marcellin P, Ahn SH, Ma X, et al. Combination of tenofovir disoproxil fumarate and peginterferon α-2a increases loss of hepatitis B surface antigen in patients with chronic hepatitis B. Gastroenterology. 2016;**150**(1):134-44.e10

Chapter 7

Advanced Hepatitis Management: Precision Medicine Integration

Nagham Nafiz Hendi, Asma Mahdi and Randa AlYafie

Abstract

Hepatitis poses a major global health challenge due to viral infections that lead to significant liver inflammation and associated morbidity and mortality. Although traditional therapies, such as antiviral medications and immunomodulatory agents, have improved patient outcomes, they are often hindered by limitations like drug resistance and varying efficacy among different populations. This chapter explores the emerging role of precision medicine in hepatitis management, focusing on tailoring treatments based on individual genetic and environmental factors. The integration of advanced technologies, including machine learning and artificial intelligence, enhances the prediction of patient responses and identifies novel biomarkers. Innovations in next-generation sequencing and mass spectrometry have also advanced our understanding of viral genetics and host responses, facilitating the development of personalized vaccines and targeted therapies. This chapter provides an overview of current and future therapeutic approaches in hepatitis management, emphasizing the transformative potential of precision medicine and technological advancements to improve patient outcomes.

Keywords: hepatitis, precision medicine, advanced treatment, antiviral drugs, functional cure

1. Introduction

Hepatitis, a significant global health issue, is marked by inflammation of the liver primarily due to viral infections, particularly hepatitis A, B, C, D, and E. Despite advances in medical science, hepatitis virus infection remains a leading cause of morbidity and mortality worldwide, affecting millions of individuals annually [1]. Current therapeutic strategies for hepatitis infection, including antiviral medications, immunomodulatory agents, and supportive care, have undoubtedly improved patient outcomes [2]. However, these treatments often have limitations such as drug resistance, adverse side effects, and varying efficacy among different populations [3].

In recent years, precision medicine has emerged as a promising approach to address these challenges. Precision medicine tailors medical treatment to the individual characteristics of each patient, considering genetic and molecular profiling, as well as environmental and lifestyle factors. This approach can potentially revolutionize hepatitis management by providing more effective and personalized therapeutic interventions [4]. Additionally, the integration of machine learning and artificial intelligence (AI) represents a new frontier in this field. AI algorithms are now being employed to predict patient responses to treatment, identify novel biomarkers, and tailor therapeutic approaches more precisely [5, 6].

Interestingly, the advent of next-generation sequencing (NGS) and mass spectrometric studies technologies has enhanced our understanding of the genetic diversity of hepatitis viruses and host responses [7, 8]. Research indicates that specific genetic variants and novel biomarkers significantly influence responses to antiviral therapies, leading to the development of personalized vaccines and more targeted treatments [9]. For example, advancements in immunotherapy are showing promise in managing chronic hepatitis B virus (HBV) [10], while new classes of direct-acting antiviral agents (DAA) are being developed to overcome resistance in hepatitis C virus (HCV), achieving sustained virologic response (SVR) rates exceeding 97% [11]. The effectiveness and ease of using DAA have made the World Health Organization's goal of eradicating HCV by 2030 a real possibility [12]. Additionally, recent advancements in clustered regularly interspaced short palindromic repeats and CRISPR-associated protein (CRISPR/Cas9) gene-editing technology offer potential for curative therapies by directly targeting viral genomes or host factors involved in viral persistence [13].

This chapter provides a comprehensive overview of current hepatitis therapies, their limitations, and how precision medicine—boosted by AI and machine learning—is reshaping treatment paradigms through advancements in genomics and bioinformatics. The discussion extends to emerging therapies, including gene editing, targeted drug delivery systems, and next-generation immunotherapies, leveraging the advancements of personalized hepatitis management and improved patient outcomes.

2. Current therapy in hepatitis infections

The management of hepatitis has evolved significantly over the past few decades, with the development of various antiviral therapies recommended for most HBV and HCV patients, except in cases of decompensated cirrhosis, pregnancy, or limited life expectancy. The primary goal is to control viral replication, reduce liver inflammation, and prevent disease progression to cirrhosis, liver failure or hepatocellular carcinoma (HCC), or liver-related mortality. Current treatment strategies can be broadly categorized into three major classes: interferons (IFNs), nucleoside/nucleotide analogues (NAs), and DAA [14, 15]. These therapies have collectively transformed hepatitis care, offering more effective and targeted approaches to managing the disease across different viral genotypes and patient populations (**Table 1**) [16].

2.1 Interferons

IFNs were among the first antiviral therapies introduced for hepatitis treatment, particularly for chronic HBV and HCV [14, 17]. These naturally occurring cytokines exhibit strong antiviral, antiproliferative, and immunomodulatory properties. Specifically, IFN-α stimulates antiviral pathways through IFN-stimulated genes and directly inhibits hepatitis viruses by suppressing viral DNA synthesis, disrupting RNA-containing core particles, accelerating their decay, and degrading pre-genomic RNA and the epigenetic of covalently closed circular DNA (cccDNA) [18, 19].

DOI: http://dx.doi.org/10.5772/intechopen.1007793

Drug Name	Class	Clinical trial ID	Clinical phase (status)	Target population	Sponsor	Mechanism of action	Efficacy/key outcomes
PEG IFN-alpha2a (Pegasys®)	Interferons	NCT00452023	II (completed)	Chronic HCV	M.D. Anderson Cancer Center	Induces antiviral state and enhances immune response	Showed significant viral suppression and SVR in combination therapy
Ribavirin	Nucleoside analogue (Antiviral)	NCT00275938	II/III (completed)	HCV, Chronic HBV	National Taiwan University Hospital	Inhibits viral RNA synthesis	Commonly used with interferons; improved SVR in HCV
Lamivudine	Nucleoside analogue	NCT02202473	IV (completed)	Chronic HBV	Southeast Universit, China	Inhibits HBV reverse transcription	Effective for reducing HBV viral load but resistance develops over time
Telbivudine	Nucleoside analogue	NCT03778567	IV (completed)	Chronic HBV	The University of Hong Kong	Selective inhibition of HBV DNA polymerase	Shows high efficacy in early-stage treatment but resistance can develop
Adefovir dipivoxil	Nucleotide analogue	NCT01205165	IV (completed)	Chronic HBV, Lamivudine-resistant patients	GlaxoSmithKline	Inhibits HBV DNA polymerase	Effective in lamivudine-resistant HBV, improves liver histology
Entecavir	Nucleoside analogue	NCT01079806	III (completed)	Chronic HBV	Bristol-Myers Squibb	Potent HBV DNA polymerase inhibitor	Strong antiviral effect, low resistance rate, high barrier to resistance
Tenofovir disoproxil fumarate (TDF)	Nucleotide analogue	NCT05286346	IV (completed)	Chronic HBV	Samjin Pharmaceutical Co., Ltd.	Inhibits HBV DNA polymerase	High efficacy in HBV, effective in lamivudine-resistant strains
Tenofovir alafenamide (TAF)	Nucleotide analogue	NCT01940341	III (completed)	Chronic HBV	Gilead Sciences	Inhibits HBV DNA polymerase with lower renal toxicity than TDF	Comparable efficacy to TDF with improved renal and bone safety
Sofosbuvir/ ledipasvir	Direct-acting antiviral	NCT02125500	II (completed)	Chronic HCV, genotype 1	ANRS, Emerging Infectious Diseases	NS5B polymerase and NS5A inhibitor	High SVR rates (over 95%), well-tolerated
Glecaprevir/ pibrentasvir	Direct-acting antiviral	NCT04903626	III (completed)	Chronic HCV, all genotypes	AbbVie	NS3/4A protease and NS5A inhibitor	Pangenotypic, very high SVR rates across genotypes, short treatment duration

Drug Name	Class	Clinical trial ID	Clinical phase (status)	Target population	Sponsor	Mechanism of action	Efficacy/key outcomes
Sofosbuvir/ velpatasvir	Direct-acting antiviral	NCT04112303	III (completed)	Chronic HCV, all genotypes	Gilead Sciences	NS5B polymerase and NS5A inhibitor	Pangenotypic efficacy, well-tolerated, high SVR rates across genotypes
Sofosbuvir/ velpatasvir/ voxilaprevir	Direct-acting antiviral	NCT04211909	III (completed)	Chronic HCV, all genotypes, treatment-experienced patients	Gilead Sciences	NS5B polymerase, NS5A inhibitor, and NS3/4A protease inhibitor	Highly effective in treatment-experienced patients, high SVR rates
Myrcludex B (bulevirtide)	Entry inhibitor	NCT02637999	I/II (completed)	Chronic HDV	Hepatera Ltd.	Inhibits HBV/HDV entry by targeting NTCP	Promising in HDV patients, reduces viral replication, well-tolerated

Data sourced from ClinicalTrials.gov provides insight into the safety and effectiveness of the current hepatitis therapies in specific patient subgroups and treatment settings. Abbreviations: NCT, ClinicalTrials.gov identifier; SVR, sustained virologic response; HBV, hepatitis B; HCV, hepatitis C; HDV, hepatitis D.

Table 1.
Summary of current therapies for hepatitis and antiviral agents.

DOI: http://dx.doi.org/10.5772/intechopen.1007793

This antiviral action is vital for infection control, enhancing innate immunity and potentially activating natural killer (NK) cells, which may help restore adaptive immune function [20]. As a result, IFN-α treatment can lower viral load and HBV surface antigen (HBsAg) levels and improve CD8 T-cell responses in sustained responders' post-treatment [21].

Standard IFN therapy had a short half-life and a modest response rate of approximately 16%, often necessitating prolonged treatment durations and frequent dosing regimens [22]. These limitations are influenced by baseline factors, such as viral genotype, viral load, sex, age, geographic location, HBsAg, and alanine aminotransferase (ALT) levels [23, 24], but their predictive value for individual patients is limited. Interestingly, research on genetic polymorphisms has yielded promising insights into individual susceptibility to IFN-α treatment. Unlike HCV, interleukin 28B (*IL-28B*) gene polymorphism has not been shown to impact IFN-α response in chronic HBV or hepatitis D [25–27]. While certain human leukocyte antigens (HLA) polymorphisms have been linked to HBV pathogenesis in specific populations [28], their correlation with IFN-α response remains inconsistent [29]. Other genetic biomarkers, such as the rs3746662 polymorphism in adenosine deaminase acting on double-stranded RNA1 (*ADAR1*) and the rs7574865 polymorphism in signal transducer and activator of transcription 4 (STAT4), have shown potential as predictors of IFN-α treatment response [30, 31]. Further study is needed to clarify the link between genetic polymorphisms and IFN response, as conclusive evidence for clinical application remains limited.

Pegylated IFN-α (Peg-IFNα) formulations have emerged as a preferred treatment for chronic hepatitis due to their extended half-life, allowing for less frequent dosing and improved patient adherence [15]. Pegylation has demonstrated effectiveness in both HBV e-antigen (HBeAg)-positive and HBeAg-negative patients, achieving significant rates of viral suppression, HBeAg seroconversion, and sustained response [32, 33]. For instance, a 48-week course of Peg-IFNα treatment in HBeAg-positive liver cirrhosis patients results in an ALT normalization, a 27% reduction in HBeAg levels, and a 25% decrease in HBV DNA [34–36]. For HBeAg-negative patients, Peg-IFNα can sustain long-term suppression of HBsAg levels for up to 3 years post-treatment, reflecting a significant SVR [37]. Despite these advances, IFN-based therapies are limited by poor patient tolerance, with notable adverse effects, such as flu-like symptoms, depression, hematological abnormalities, and thyroid dysfunction. These issues can lead to a high rate of treatment discontinuation and contraindicate Peg-IFNα use in patients with decompensated or severe compensated cirrhosis and during pregnancy [3, 24].

Ribavirin, an oral guanosine analog, was introduced to enhance interferon (IFN) therapy, leading to reduced relapse rates and modest improvements in cure rates, reaching 41% for genotype 1 and nearly 75% for other genotypes [38]. It remained the standard therapy until 2011, though its effectiveness varied, showing greater success in HBeAg-positive patients, hindered by significant toxicity, especially in advanced liver disease [39]. For severe cases or acute-on-chronic liver failure caused by the hepatitis E virus, ribavirin is recommended [40], with a 12-week monotherapy course prescribed for persistent replication beyond 3 months [41]. Although generally well tolerated, ribavirin can cause hemolytic anemia, particularly in patients with renal impairment due to its renal excretion [42]. It is contraindicated in individuals with a creatinine clearance below 50 mL/min and should be avoided in pregnant women due to its teratogenic effects [43].

Given the limited proportion of sustained responders, tailoring treatment to individual patients is essential for optimizing IFN-based therapy. For instance, in HBeAg-negative patients, the lack of HBsAg decline after 12 weeks of therapy predicts non-response, especially in genotype D patients [44]. Integrating baseline factors, like viral genotype, age, and ALT levels, with on-treatment predictors, such as HBV-RNA and HBsAg kinetics, could enhance personalized treatment and long-term outcomes.

2.2 Nucleoside/nucleotide analogues

NAs have become a cornerstone in the treatment of chronic HBV [15], and to a lesser extent, HCV [14]. Currently available NAs, include lamivudine, adefovir dipivoxil, entecavir, telbivudine, tenofovir disoproxil fumarate (TDF), and tenofovir alafenamide, target viral polymerase to inhibit replication. They integrate into hepatitis viral DNA during replication, which causes premature chain termination and blocks the reverse transcription of RNA to DNA [45].

Lamivudine was the first nucleoside analogue to significantly inhibit viral replication, but its clinical utility was constrained by variable effectiveness and high resistance rates [46]. While about 40% of patients experienced HBeAg suppression after 3 years of treatment, resistance rates could reach 20% within the first year and escalate to 70% after 5 years, leading to viral breakthroughs and potential liver failure [45, 47]. Similarly, resistance with telbivudine can reach up to 22% in HBeAg-positive and 9% in HBeAg-negative patients [45, 48]. Moreover, lamivudine and telbivudine can cause mitochondrial toxicity, including myopathies and neuropathies [49], although lactic acidosis from lamivudine is rare [50].

Second-generation NAs, like entecavir, TDF, and tenofovir alafenamide, are highly potent antiviral agents with a strong resistance barrier, making them the preferred first-line treatments for chronic HBV [15]. These analogues inhibit HBV-DNA synthesis by competing with essential nucleotides, which reduces new hepatocyte infections, dilutes the intrahepatic cccDNA pool, and decreases its transcription. This cumulative effect gradually declines viral markers and modulates immune responses, potentially enabling some patients to control hepatitis infection without ongoing therapy. After around 5 years of treatment, 94–96% of HBeAg-positive and 95–99% of HBeAg-negative patients achieve undetectable HBV DNA levels [51]. TDF also demonstrates notable HBeAg loss in 49–53% of patients and a cumulative HBsAg loss of 11% [52].

Long-term NA treatment, well-tolerated oral medications, effectively suppresses viral replication over extended periods. Despite advancements, sustained therapy is often necessary due to the persistence of cccDNA, which can lead to viral reactivation after treatment discontinuation [53]. This extended use can result in resistance in up to 30% of patients, as incomplete viral suppression allows continued virion production and new hepatocyte infection [54]. Additionally, these treatments may cause nephrotoxicity and reduced bone mineral density [55]. Tenofovir alafenamide has emerged as a promising alternative, offering lower risks of renal and bone complications with improved potency and efficacy in normalizing ALT levels [56].

Recent strategies to overcome the limitations of monotherapies involve combining NAs with other agents, such as the virus entry inhibitor Myrcludex-B, which enhances antiviral activity by preventing intrahepatic viral spread and new infections [57]. This combination suggests that residual infective virions contribute to cccDNA persistence and transcription, as NAs do not impact cccDNA stability or transcription, leading to the ongoing production of viral proteins and pre-genomes [58]. Additionally, combining PEG-IFNα with entecavir has shown more promising outcomes than with lamivudine or telbivudine, with significant reductions in HBeAg and HBsAg levels.

The combination of PEG-IFNα with entecavir or TDF may also offer more sustained suppression of viral markers, although efficacy may vary with hepatitis B virus genotypes, particularly for genotypes C and D [59].

NAs may be discontinued in HBeAg-positive chronic HBV patients without cirrhosis after achieving undetectable HBV-DNA and HBeAg seroconversion, followed by 6–12 months consolidation period [60]. Anti-hepatitis B e-antigen (Anti-Hb) seroconversion typically persists in over 85% of patients for at least 2 years post-discontinuation. However, HBsAg clearance is the preferred endpoint for discontinuation in HBeAg-negative patients, though clearance rates remain low. Serum viral DNA often reappears within 6 months after discontinuation, with relapse rates of 35% at 6 months and 55% at 2 years [61]. Notably, lower HBsAg levels at discontinuation correlate with higher rates of sustained virological response [60]. The current European Association for the Study of the Liver (EASL) guidelines recommend discontinuing NAs only in non-cirrhotic patients with at least 3 years of virological suppression, with close monitoring for potential relapse [15].

2.3 Direct-acting antiviral agents

The advent of DAA has revolutionized the treatment landscape for HCV, achieving SVR rates exceeding 97% with shorter treatment durations, around 8 to 12 weeks, and fewer side effects compared to previous regimens [62]. Contemporary oral DAA target essential viral non-structural proteins (NS) necessary for replication, specifically NS3/4A protease, NS5A, and NS5B polymerases. These antiviral agents are categorized based on their molecular targets, such as protease inhibitors (ending in "-previr"), NS5A inhibitors (ending in "-asvir"), and NS5B polymerase inhibitors (ending in "-buvir"). Despite these advances, about 4–5% of patients may not achieve viral eradication due to factors like poor adherence, relapse, advanced liver disease, or resistance mutations [63]. HCV's rapid evolution can create resistance-associated variants, mainly in the NS5A region, but also in NS3 and NS5B [64].

Pangenotypic DAA combinations—such as sofosbuvir/velpatasvir (Epclusa), glecaprevir/pibrentasvir (Mavyret), sofosbuvir/ledipasvir (Harvoni), and sofosbuvir/velpatasvir/voxilaprevir (Vosevi)—are now the standard of care for treating HCV across all genotypes [14]. These regimens are effective even in patients with advanced liver disease and other comorbidities, with treatment choice guided by genotype, renal function, and concurrent medications [62]. However, protease inhibitors, primarily excreted through the liver, are contraindicated in patients with decompensated cirrhosis, those co-infected with human immunodeficiency viruses (HIV), or individuals who have undergone liver transplantation [65]. Additionally, sofosbuvir, a nucleoside NS5B inhibitor, is avoided in those with significant renal impairment [66].

Traditionally, treating acute HCV—defined as the first 6 months post-infection—was challenging and often required Peg-IFNα if viral replication persisted beyond 12 weeks. However, DAA now demonstrate effectiveness in the early stages of infection, particularly in high-risk populations, such as injection drug users, men who have sex with men, and individuals with HIV. In these groups, DAA can reduce morbidity, mortality, and transmission risk before the disease progresses to chronicity [67]. The EASL recommends an 8-week course of sofosbuvir/velpatasvir or glecaprevir/pibrentasvir for recently acquired HCV, although post-exposure prophylaxis with DAA is not advised without confirmed HCV transmission [14].

Liver transplantation remains a vital intervention for patients with HCV-related decompensated cirrhosis or HCC, despite a notable reduction in transplant demand due to the effectiveness of DAA [68]. Before the introduction of DAA, nearly all HCV-positive liver transplant recipients experienced recurrent infection post-transplantation, leading to severe complications such as fibrosis, recurrent cirrhosis, and fibrosing cholestatic hepatitis, with significantly reduced survival rates compared to HCV-negative recipients [69]. DAA have since dramatically enhanced the management of HCV in liver transplant candidates, improving overall survival and reducing graft rejection by preventing recurrence or achieving SVR when administered pre- or post-transplant [70]. This advancement extends to other solid organ transplants, making organ donation from HCV-positive donors more feasible and reducing waitlist mortality and healthcare costs [71]. HCV-negative recipients of HCV-positive organs are typically treated with DAA, either prophylactically or reactively upon detection of HCV RNA [72], with early studies showing high rates of SVR and graft survival outcomes [71].

While the simplicity of pangenotypic regimens marks a significant advancement, the high cost of DAA limits accessibility, particularly in low- and middle-income countries [73]. Ongoing concerns include resistance-associated variants, persistence of HCV RNA post-SVR, fibrosing cholestatic hepatitis, drug interactions, and challenges in treating co-infected or advanced liver disease patients. Some studies also report reduced efficacy of regimens like Vosevi in certain genotypes with cirrhosis [74]. Patients with advanced fibrosis remain at risk for liver complications and HCC, necessitating continued surveillance even after achieving SVR [75]. Although early fears suggested DAA could increase HCC recurrence by disrupting immune surveillance of pre-existing tumors, recent evidence refutes this risk, confirming SVR's importance for improving liver function and long-term survival [76]. The timing of DAA initiation in HCV-positive HCC patients remains controversial, requiring adherence to updated guidelines to optimize outcomes and minimize risks [77].

3. Advanced therapy in hepatitis infections

The management landscape for hepatitis continues to evolve as medical science advances toward eradicating this global health threat. Notable advancement has been made with the new therapeutic technologies and translational research, offering new hope for patients, particularly those unresponsive to traditional treatments. One such breakthrough is the approval of bulevirtide in Europe for hepatitis D virus (HDV), which provides a targeted approach for patients who do not respond to interferon-based therapies [78]. Since HDV relies on HBV for replication, patients with HDV are often treated with antiviral therapies aimed at reducing HBV levels, such as tenofovir or entecavir, which indirectly help in controlling HDV [79].

The development of advanced treatments for HBV and HCV is increasingly recognized as a necessity, drawing significant attention from both researchers and clinicians. Chronic HBV and HCV pose significant challenges that can progress to severe liver diseases, such as cirrhosis and HCC [80]. Despite the availability of antiviral treatments, the management of chronic hepatitis infections remains difficult due to the limitations of current therapies. These treatments may cause significant side effects and safety issues, and require lifelong use due to the risk of viral rebound upon discontinuation [81]. Additionally, the high global burden of chronic HBV and HCV infections, affecting millions of people worldwide, underscores the need for more effective, long-term therapeutic strategies.

One of the key challenges in treating HCV lies in the diversity of viral genotypes, which complicates therapeutic development. Recent advancements in DAA have significantly improved treatment efficacy and tolerability with broad-spectrum efficacy across genotypes. However, DAA remain expensive and even after a successful treatment, patients are vulnerable to reinfection if exposed to the virus again [82]. Given these ongoing challenges, the research focus has shifted toward innovative therapeutic strategies, including gene therapy, immunomodulatory approaches, and novel vaccine development. These advancements hold the promise of providing more durable, tailored treatment for patients with chronic infections, particularly those inadequately served by current modalities. Several novel agents are under development for chronic hepatitis infections as detailed in **Table 2** highlighting the latest advancements, drawn from ongoing clinical trials.

3.1 Innovations in gene therapy

Gene therapy is emerging as a promising strategy, particularly for HBV. Central to this effort is the episomal cccDNA, an HBV replication intermediate that forms a minichromosome in the hepatocyte nucleus. A few copies of cccDNA can cause infection to rebound after treatment cessation through producing HBsAg in the bloodstream [83]. Current research focuses on gene therapies that silence cccDNA to achieve a functional or complete cure for HBV.

RNA interference (RNAi) offers a promising approach for treating chronic HBV by using small interfering RNA (siRNA) to target and suppress HBV mRNA selectively. A key advantage of siRNA therapies is their ability to target overlapping regions of the HBV genome, such as the X region, allowing a single siRNA to knock down all HBV transcripts [84]. However, efficient delivery to hepatocytes remains a challenge. This has been addressed by conjugating siRNA with ligands such as a tri-antennary N-acetyl galactosamine (GalNAc), which binds to the asialoglycoprotein receptor on hepatocytes and facilitates rapid endocytosis [85]. Early siRNA therapies encountered issues like off-target effects and hepatotoxicity. However, the modified siRNA VIR-2218, with improved stabilization, has shown a favorable safety profile and significant reductions in HBsAg levels, indicating its potential in future chronic HBV treatments [86].

Recent advancements emphasize the importance of co-delivery and optimized encapsulation systems. Researchers have developed a broad-spectrum siRNA encapsulated in a targeted lipid nanoparticle (tLNP) with 98.55% genotypic coverage. This system led to significant reductions in viral antigens and DNA levels in mouse models. Moreover, the co-delivery of siRNA with *IL-2* mRNA further improved viral suppression, presenting a promising dual-modality therapeutic strategy [84]. Although RNAi therapies aim for a functional cure by reducing viral replication and many RNAi candidates have progressed to clinical trials, they often require repeated dosing and are used in combination with other treatments. This is where gene-editing technologies offer the potential to provide precise and permanent alterations to the viral genome that could eliminate its replication.

In addition to siRNA, other RNAi modalities, such as short hairpin RNA (shRNA) and gene-editing technologies like zinc-finger nucleases (ZFNs) and transcription activator-like effector nucleases (TALENs), have demonstrated potential in disrupting viral hepatitis DNA. For instance, lentiviral vectors have been used to express single, double, or triple shRNA cassettes targeting conserved viral sequences and host factors critical for HCV replication, without causing significant cytotoxicity [87].

Drug name	Class	Clinical trial ID	Clinical phase (Status)	Target population	Sponsor	Mechanism of action	Efficacy/key outcomes
AHB-137	siRNA	NCT06550128	I (recruiting)	Chronic HBV	Ausper Biopharma Co., Ltd.	Silencing HBV RNA via RNA interference	Reduction in HBV viral load; improvement in liver function tests
TT-034	siRNA	NCT01899092	I/II (completed)	Chronic HBV	Tacere Therapeutics, Inc.	Targeting HBV RNA for degradation	Significant decrease in HBV DNA levels; serological response
JNJ-73763989	siRNA	NCT05005507	II (terminated)	Chronic HBV	Janssen Research & Development, LLC	RNA interference targeting HBV transcripts	Notable safety concerns; reduced HBV RNA levels
RG6346 (DCR-HBVS)	siRNA	NCT03772249	I (completed)	Chronic HBV	Dicerna Pharmaceuticals, Inc., Novo Nordisk	Silencing HBV replication via RNA interference	Viral suppression; enhanced immune response
RO7020531	IMA	NCT02956850	I (completed)	Chronic HBV	Hoffmann-La Roche	Stimulates immune response to viral antigens by activating TLR7 agonist	Enhanced T-cell activation; reduction in viral antigen levels
Durvalumab (MEDI 4736)	IMA	NCT04294498	II (active, not recruiting)	Chronic HBV	National Taiwan University Hospital	Immune checkpoint inhibitor targeting PD-L1	Increased overall survival; improved response rates
VIR-3434	IMA	NCT04423393	I (completed)	Chronic HBV	Vir Biotechnology, Inc.	Monoclonal antibody neutralizing HBV surface antigen	Decrease in HBV surface antigen; improved immune response
Hepalatide	IMA	NCT06505928	II (not yet recruiting)	Chronic HBV	Shanghai HEP Pharmaceutical Co., Ltd.	Enhances immune response to clear HBV-infected T-cells	Potential improvement in serological markers
RO7049389 (CpAM)	IMA	NCT02952924	I (completed)	Chronic HBV	Hoffmann-La Roche	Core protein allosteric modulator, inhibiting HBV capsid assembly	Viral load reduction; tolerability profile
YS-HBV-002	IMA	NCT06162299	I (not yet recruiting)	Chronic HBV	Yisheng Biopharma (Singapore) Pte. Ltd.	Induces immune response to target HBV	Early immunogenicity results expected

DOI: http://dx.doi.org/10.5772/intechopen.1007793

Drug name	Class	Clinical trial ID	Clinical phase (Status)	Target population	Sponsor	Mechanism of action	Efficacy/key outcomes
FP-02.2	Therapeutic vaccine	NCT02496897	I (completed)	Chronic HBV	Altimmune, Inc.	Activates immune response to prevent HBV reactivation	Immunogenic response; improved patient outcomes
TherVacB	Therapeutic vaccine	NCT06513286	I/II (not yet recruiting)	Chronic HBV	Michael Hoelscher	Therapeutic vaccination to eliminate HBV-infected cells	Expected improvement in HBV clearance; safety profile analysis
BRII-179	Therapeutic vaccine	NCT06491563	II (not yet recruiting)	Chronic HBV	Brii Biosciences Limited	Stimulates immune system to attack HBV-infected cells	Enhanced immune response; potential reduction in viral load
Hecolin	Therapeutic vaccine	NCT06306196	II (not yet recruiting)	HEV	International Vaccine Institute	Targets prevention of HEV infections	Efficacy in reducing HEV incidence; seroconversion rates
JNJ-64300535	Therapeutic vaccine	NCT03463369	I (completed)	Chronic HBV	Janssen Research & Development, LLC	Immune response against HBV-infected T-cells	Improved serological markers; overall safety profile

Data sourced from ClinicalTrials.gov provides an overview of advanced treatments in clinical trials for hepatitis. Abbreviaitons: siRNAs, small interfering RNAs; HBV, hepatitis B virus; HEV, hepatitis E virus; CpAMs, core protein allosteric modulators; NCT, ClinicalTrials.gov identifier; TLR7, toll-like receptor 7; PD-L1, programmed death-ligand 1; IMA, immunomodulatory agent.

Table 2.
Summary of emerging advanced therapies for hepatitis.

ZFNs are engineered proteins combining DNA-binding abilities with nuclease activity for genome editing. By linking multiple Zinc-finger domains with a FokI nuclease, ZFNs can create site-specific double-strand breaks in DNA, enabling precise genome modifications [88]. Studies have shown ZFNs' ability to disrupt HBV DNA and reduce viral replication, but most research has been limited to *in vitro* models, and concerns about off-target effects and cytotoxicity require further *in vivo* investigation [89].

Newer gene-editing technologies, like TALENs, have offered improved accuracy and safety profiles. Derived from Xanthomonas bacteria, TALENs function as dimers, utilizing the FokI nuclease for DNA cleavage. Compared to ZFNs, TALENs exhibit higher specificity, lower off-target effects, and reduced cytotoxicity, making them versatile tools against chronic viral infections like HBV [90]. In cell cultures and animal models, TALENs have effectively suppressed HBV replication by reducing HBsAg levels. By targeting both core and surface open reading frames, TALENs have shown robust antiviral effects, significantly reducing viral particles *in vivo* [91]. However, their efficacy is time-dependent, and results vary across different HBV genotypes and target sites. While TALENs have had some success in disrupting cccDNA, more research is needed to optimize their targeting of this critical viral reservoir.

The emergence of more precise gene-editing tools like CRISPR has overshadowed ZFN and TALEN technologies, although these earlier tools still offer a foundation for future antiviral strategies. The CRISPR/Cas system is a revolutionary third-generation gene-editing technology that uses guide RNA (gRNA) to direct the Cas protein to specific genomic sites, enhancing accuracy and efficiency [92]. In HBV research, CRISPR technology has shown promise by targeting regions of the viral genome with single guide RNAs (sgRNAs). Targeting the HBV X gene, for instance, has led to reductions in cccDNA, replication intermediates, HBsAg, and HBcAg [93]. In transgenic mouse models, CRISPR/Cas9, delivered via adeno-associated virus serotype 8 (AAV8), significantly reduced HBV core protein expression in the liver and lowered serum HBsAg levels, highlighting its antiviral potential [94].

Despite significant advancements in gene and RNA-based therapies, effective delivery of these synthetic nucleic acid effectors remains a significant challenge, and they face difficulty penetrating lipid membranes. The success of these therapies depends on developing advanced, functional delivery systems for *in vivo* use. Ongoing research is focused on next-generation delivery technologies and optimizing siRNA design to improve intracellular efficiency and extend therapeutic duration [95]. Continued innovation in delivery systems, combined with the refinement of therapeutic nucleic acids, offers great potential for overcoming delivery challenges, minimizing off-target effects, and advancing safer, more effective treatments—bringing us closer to functional cures for chronic diseases like hepatitis infection [12].

3.2 Targeted immunomodulatory therapies

In addition to gene therapies, immunomodulatory treatments are emerging as powerful tools for combating hepatitis infections. These therapies enhance the innate and adaptive immune responses, enabling the body to better fight the virus. By boosting immune activity or restoring exhausted immune cells, immunomodulatory therapies can complement gene therapies, offering a multifaceted approach to managing or potentially curing chronic hepatitis infections. Toll-like receptors (TLRs) are pivotal in the innate immune defense, recognizing pathogen-associated molecular patterns (PAMPs) and initiating cytokine production through various signaling pathways. Specifically, TLR-7 and TLR-8 agonists help induce IFN production, activate

IFN-stimulated genes (ISGs), and trigger signaling cascades like JAK/STAT. The TLR-7 agonist GS-9620 has demonstrated the ability to suppress HBV through type I IFN induction in human hepatocyte cell lines, though it does not reduce cccDNA [96]. However, when combined with the TLR-7 agonist RO7020531 with a capsid assembly modulator, HBV DNA and HBsAg levels were significantly reduced in a mouse model [97]. In healthy human volunteers, TLR-7 agonists induced IFN-alpha and ISG expression, though further studies are needed to evaluate their efficacy in combination with other antiviral agents [98].

Recent advancements in chronic HBV therapies have focused on enhancing innate immunity. Retinoic acid-inducible gene-I (RIG-I) agonists, such as Inarigivir (SB 9200), activate immune pathways, leading to reduced HBV DNA and RNA levels. Clinical trials have shown that 22% of patients experienced HBsAg reduction, and higher doses of Inarigivir combined with tenofovir are currently under investigation [99]. Additionally, checkpoint inhibitors, such as the PD-1 inhibitor nivolumab, aim to restore T-cell function. Trials have demonstrated significant HBsAg reduction in some patients, and cytotoxic T-lymphocyte-associated protein 4 (CTLA-4) blockade has also shown potential in improving immune responses against HBV [100]. These therapies represent promising steps toward more effective treatment strategies for chronic HBV.

Among the most innovative strategies for treating chronic HBV are T-cell-based therapies. In chronic HBV patients, T-cell exhaustion often impairs immune function, hindering effective viral control [101]. One promising approach involves generating functional HBV-specific T cells from patients and re-infusing them to overcome immune energy. Evidence from bone marrow and organ transplant cases suggests that adoptive transfer of engineered antigen-specific T cells can control HBV. These T cells, engineered via viral vectors to recognize HBV antigens, have shown encouraging results in HBV transgenic mice [102]. However, challenges such as the large-scale production of engineered T cells and complex regulatory and technological hurdles remain barriers to their widespread clinical application.

3.3 Advances in therapeutic vaccination

Therapeutic vaccines for chronic HBV have been explored to modulate the adaptive immune system and overcome immune exhaustion. In early attempts, an antigen-antibody complex vaccine (HBsAg-HBIG) with alum as an adjuvant (YIC) was tested to overcome immune tolerance. While the YIC vaccine initially showed promise, overstimulation led to immune fatigue, reducing its efficacy and underscoring the need to optimize immunization strategies [103]. Recent approaches, like ABX-203 (HeberNasvac), a vaccine containing HBsAg and HBcAg, have shown promise in clinical trials, achieving better viral load reduction and HBeAg seroconversion compared to Peg-IFNα [104]. Vector-based vaccines, like GS-4774 and TG-1050, which use viral vectors to encode HBV antigens and enhance T-cell activation, have demonstrated strong immune responses. However, these vaccines have yet to significantly reduce HBsAg levels in treated patients [105, 106]. Breaking immune tolerance remains a critical challenge in chronic HBV infection. For example, TG-1050 has demonstrated safety and immunogenicity, but pre-existing adenoviral immunity can limit its effectiveness, even though it has stimulated anti-HBV immune responses and activated cytotoxic functions in animal models [106]. Despite their limitations, combining these vaccines with antiviral agents or improving delivery methods may boost their therapeutic potential for HBV treatment.

Recent advancements in HCV vaccine development are focused on overcoming past challenges, such as the virus's high genetic variability, lack of suitable animal models, and limited understanding of protective immune responses. Approaches like mRNA vaccines offer rapid testing of potential candidates and aim to stimulate strong, multi-specific cellular immune responses, including helper and cytotoxic T cells, along with high-titer, long-lasting, cross-reactive anti-envelope antibodies. HCV envelope glycoproteins, particularly E1 and E2, have become promising vaccine targets [107]. New approaches to vaccine design emphasize the identification of neutralizing antibodies associated with viral clearance by creating epitopes, like E2, to stimulate potent antiviral antibodies, such as HC33.1 and AP33, which have shown broad and robust HCV neutralization in experimental models [108].

Another promising strategy uses dendritic cells (DC) expressing HCV-derived core or NS3 antigens to activate autologous T cells, leading to cytokine production and strong immune responses [109]. Additionally, GS-9620, a small molecule agonist targeting DC receptor toll-like receptor 7 (TLR7), was developed to activate DCs, functioning as innate immune-like vaccines [96]. Although GS-9620 did not significantly reduce HBsAg levels in clinical trials, it enhanced HBV-specific T cells and NK cell responses in patients receiving NUC treatment [110]. Another example, GI-13020 (GS-4774), a heat-killed recombinant yeast expressing an HBx-HBs-HBc chimeric protein, elicited both CD4+ and CD8+ T-cell responses with acceptable initial tolerability. However, in Phase 2 trials, it did not lead to significant reductions in HBsAg levels [111].

A recent study highlights the vital role of adjuvants in boosting vaccine efficacy by enhancing innate immunity. Researchers examined gene expression in naive individuals vaccinated with hepatitis B surface antigen alongside various adjuvants, identifying a core innate immune signature that emerged after the second dose. This signature included the positive regulation of INF-related responses and activation of innate immune cells, which correlated with stronger antibody production. Notably, the adjuvant AS01B was especially effective in generating this inflammatory signature after the first dose, indicating that its success may depend more on its ability to elicit consistent immune responses across individuals rather than the specific receptors or pathways it targets [112].

While therapeutic vaccines hold great promise in strengthening immune response against chronic hepatitis infections, several challenges remain. One significant limitation is the variability in individual immune responses, which can affect the overall efficacy of the vaccine [113]. Genetic background, pre-existing immunity, and co-infections can influence patient responses to vaccination [114]. Additionally, the risk of adverse effects, including autoimmune reactions, poses a concern that requires careful consideration in vaccine design and implementation [115]. Addressing these challenges is essential for successfully integrating therapeutic vaccines into treatment protocols for chronic hepatitis infections.

4. Precision medicine integration in hepatitis infections

Precision medicine, an approach that tailors medical treatment to the individual characteristics of each patient, has revolutionized the management of infectious diseases [5]. Laboratory diagnostics for viral hepatitis focus on detecting viral proteins, nucleic acids, antibodies, and biochemical markers produced in response to infection [116]. Molecular techniques, such as nucleic acid testing (NAT) through polymerase chain reaction (PCR) and microbial protein analysis via mass spectrometry, are increasingly favored for their superior sensitivity and specificity in detecting pathogens.

While serologic tests remain the standard for diagnosing viral hepatitis, NAT methods may complement them in certain cases [117]. Rapid diagnostic tests (RDTs), which offer quick, cost-effective detection of HBsAg in non-laboratory settings, are becoming a valuable quantitative immunochromatographic tool for widespread screening [118, 119]. However, selecting the most appropriate diagnostic approach requires a thorough understanding of viral transmission, disease progression, viral kinetics, and testing limitations [117].

In the context of hepatitis infections, precision medicine leverages advanced technologies, such as next-generation sequencing, pharmacogenomics, and mass spectrometry, to enhance diagnostic precision, optimize therapeutic strategies, and improve patient outcomes. By integrating genetic, environmental, and lifestyle factors, this approach deepens the understanding of host-pathogen interactions in hepatitis, ultimately advancing the goals of individualized care and disease elimination [12].

4.1 Advancements in next-generation gene sequencing

Next-generation sequencing (NGS) has emerged as a transformative tool in clinical virology by providing significantly enhanced sensitivity compared to traditional Sanger sequencing, particularly in detecting drug resistance mutations, mixed genotypes, and viral quasi-species, including minor circulating variants [120]. Second-generation sequencing techniques have proven particularly adept at identifying and quantifying viral mutations and recombination events [121], while third-generation sequencing enables full-genome analysis [122]. NGS has also been pivotal in discovering novel viruses, including arenaviruses, Zika, and Ebola [123–125]. Additionally, it has facilitated the characterization of viral populations in animal and human hosts within natural environments [126, 127].

In hepatitis, NGS has significantly advanced the identification of HBV genotype mixtures, particularly in regions such as the preS and the 5′ end of the HBV X gene [128]. Despite its numerous advantages, a major limitation of NGS is the overwhelming amount of data produced, requiring advanced bioinformatic tools for proper interpretation [129]. While third-generation sequencing holds promise for comprehensive genome exploration, its clinical applicability remains hindered by higher sequencing error rates [122]. Additionally, there are challenges in variant interpretation across diverse clinical settings, which can complicate hepatitis diagnosis and prognosis [130].

4.2 Precision pharmacogenomics

Pharmacogenomics has revolutionized the personalization of drug prescriptions by exploring how individual genetic variations influence drug response, focusing primarily on pharmacokinetics and pharmacodynamics [131]. The main goal is to optimize therapeutic efficacy and minimize adverse drug reactions by tailoring treatments and risk assessments to an individual's genetic profile [132, 133]. This field incorporates data from the Human Genome Project and other genetic databases to advance genomic-based therapies and drug discovery [134]. Genome-wide association studies (GWAS) remain the gold standard for identifying pharmacogenomic associations, despite the high cost and labor intensity associated with these studies [135–137].

GWAS primarily focus on identifying single nucleotide polymorphisms (SNPs) that influence the development and progression of liver diseases, including hepatitis and hereditary liver disorders. These SNPs contribute to differences in immune responses among HBV-infected patients, which can range from asymptomatic infections to severe conditions such as cirrhosis and end-stage HCC [138]. Several studies have identified polymorphisms in the HLA complex, which regulates innate and adaptive immunity during infections, as being associated with varying clinical outcomes in chronic HBV and HCV infections, influencing both viral clearance and progression to chronic stages [139]. Additionally, various *HLA* polymorphisms linked to the response to the HBV vaccine and infection persistence have been highlighted by several studies [140, 141]. Notably, SNPs within the *HLA-DPA1* (rs3077), *HLA-DPB1* (rs9277535), and *HLA-DQ* (rs2856718 and rs7453920) have been linked to chronic HBV outcomes, especially in Asian and American populations [135, 142, 143]. Protective HLA alleles, such as *DQB106:03:01 and DRB1*13:01:01, have also been identified in Romanian populations, underscoring the geographical and ethnic variability in genetic susceptibility to HBV [144]. Beyond HLA polymorphisms, other genetic variants, such as those in *ZNF208*, have been implicated in HBV pathogenesis [145].

Host genetic factors, including *IL28B*, *interferon-λ3*, *interferon-λ4*, *IL-12*, *IL-10*, and *TLRs*, are strongly associated with treatment outcomes and disease progression [146–161]. The *IL28B* genotype has been a significant predictor of SVR in HCV patients undergoing treatment with Peg-IFNα and ribavirin. Variants, such as rs12979860, have shown a strong association with treatment success, particularly in Caucasian individuals, where those with the CC genotype achieve SVR at a rate six times higher than those with the CT or TT genotypes [162–165]. Furthermore, genetic variants in *TLRs*, such as rs3775290 "CC" genotype, have been linked to the severity of liver fibrosis, cirrhosis risk, and HCV treatment outcomes by modulating immune responses through inflammatory cytokine production [166, 167]. The role of genetic polymorphisms in interferon lambda (*IFNL*) genes in viral clearance and liver disease progression further supports the importance of genetic profiling in managing HBV and HCV infections [168]. Interferon regulatory factors (IRFs), essential transcription factors in immune cell development, have also been associated with protection against HCV infection and cirrhosis by reducing the frequency of the IRF3 "AG" genotype [169, 170]. Additionally, emerging evidence directly links microRNAs (miRNAs) with HCV infection and HCC development, emphasizing the importance of investigating their regulatory roles in disease progression [171, 172].

Despite the promise of pharmacogenomics, the field encounters several challenges, primarily the high costs of large-scale GWAS and the substantial expenses related to data storage and analysis. These financial burdens also raise ethical concerns, especially around patient privacy and potential impacts on insurance coverage [173]. Additionally, genetic findings often vary across ethnic populations, and the absence of standardized workflows for variant interpretation further limits the universal applicability of pharmacogenomic insights in clinical practice [174]. Although debates persist on the impact of genetic polymorphisms in HBV outcomes, the genetic findings are anticipated to improve individualized risk assessments and vaccination approaches, aiding in the effort to eliminate hepatitis infections as a global health threat by 2030 [12].

4.3 Integration of mass spectrometry

Mass spectrometry (MS) has become an indispensable tool in virology, enabling detailed analysis of viral capsid proteins, viral mutants, post-translational modifications, and intact viruses [175, 176], advancing antiviral drug development and evaluation [177]. Compared to NGS, MS offers a cost-effective, user-friendly alternative and has been successfully applied to genetic typing, the detection of viral biomarkers, and advancing antiviral drug development and evaluation [178]. MS applications in virology have evolved two main paths: the development of specialized techniques for measuring viral physicochemical properties and the adaptation of proteomics and interactomics approaches to address virology-specific challenges.

MS techniques such as charge-detection MS (CDMS), ion mobility spectrometry (IMS), and gas-phase electrophoretic mobility molecular analysis (GEMMA) have proven valuable in analyzing high molecular weight molecules, including viruses [179]. Adaptations of electrospray ionization-MS (ESI-MS) and matrix-assisted laser desorption/ionization mass spectrometry (MALDI-MS) have demonstrated effectiveness in detecting HBV and HCV, identifying all eight HBV genotypes [179]. When combined with multiplex PCR, MALDI-MS has been used to analyze multiple human enteric viruses, including hepatitis E virus [180]. The MALDI-MS coupled with time-of-flight (TOF) analysis offers high sensitivity and throughput, facilitating the mass screening of HBV patients undergoing lamivudine treatment [181].

MS-based proteomics has also shown that alterations in the cellular proteome, such as fatty acid chain modifications, play a role in preventing the progression of chronic HBV infection to HCC [182, 183]. Additionally, LC-MS-based metabolomic profiling has enabled the identification of metabolic biomarkers that differentiate chronic HBV from liver cirrhosis and HCC, improving early diagnosis and personalized treatment approaches [184, 185]. For HCV, gas chromatography-MS (GC-MS) analysis has linked altered glucose metabolism and branched-chain amino acids to hepatocellular damage and hyperglycemia in HCV-infected patients [186]. Furthermore, GC-MS-based metabolomic studies have identified biomarkers predictive of HCC recurrence, combining glutamate with aspartate as well as glycerol with proline, offering new avenues for monitoring disease progression before and after treatment [187].

Despite its broad applications, MS faces limitations in sensitivity and specificity when applied to complex viral populations. The integration of MS into clinical practice requires further validation to establish standardized workflows for viral detection and analysis [173].

5. Future perspectives on viral hepatitis therapy

Innovations in precision medicine, particularly through the integration of gene editing technologies, machine learning, and AI, hold immense promise for advancing hepatitis treatment (**Figure 1**). These advancements potentially eradicate viral hepatitis by directly modifying viral DNA, improving upon current therapies that only suppress viral replication [188–190]. Multi-omics analyses and GWAS also offer deeper insights into viral-host interactions, paving the way for personalized antiviral strategies, new drug targets and early detection biomarkers [190, 191].

As pharmacogenomic approaches evolve, the development of polygenic risk scores may further tailor treatments [131], especially for patients with comorbidities like liver cirrhosis or HCC. Immunotherapies, including engineered T-cell therapies and therapeutic vaccines, could boost the immune system's ability to clear persistent infections and support global eradication efforts for chronic hepatitis in the near future [12]. However, challenges in clinical implementation persist due to genetic

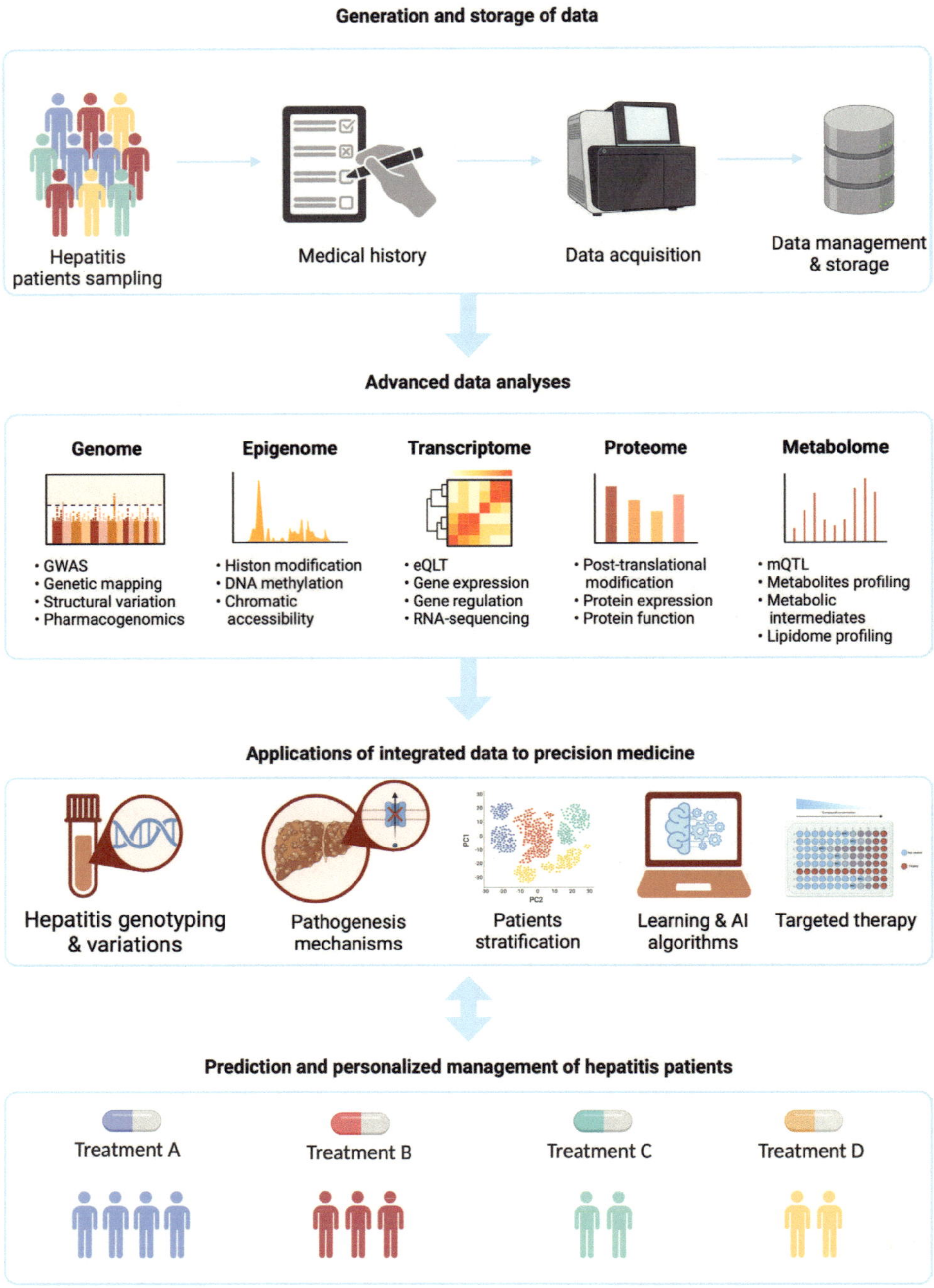

Figure 1.
Advanced data integration in hepatitis subtyping and precision medicine. This workflow demonstrates the use of advanced technologies—multi-omics, machine learning, and artificial intelligence —to refine hepatitis subtyping and personalize treatment strategies. It emphasizes identifying high-risk patients and ensuring high-quality data for analysis. Machine learning integrates these data sets to enable precise diagnostics, novel therapeutic target discovery, and customized treatments, improving patient outcomes. Abbreviations: GWAS, genome-wide association studies; eQTL, expression quantitative trait loci; mQTL, methylation quantitative trait loci; AI, artificial intelligence. Generated using BioRender.

diversity, limited sample sizes, and complex gene-drug interactions. Addressing these barriers requires interdisciplinary collaboration and the application of machine learning and AI to analyze patient-specific data, such as viral genotypes and immune responses, to improve therapeutic precision [131, 188]. Advancements in point-of-care genetic testing and early intervention strategies promise more timely and personalized treatments, making precision medicine increasingly effective in hepatitis management [192].

In this chapter, we present an advanced strategy for diagnosing and treating hepatitis patients following the latest clinical recommendations (**Figure 2**) [14, 15]. Genomic screening to detect patient-specific genetic mutations is highly recommended before starting treatment, especially for those with key pathogenic mutations. It is also important to provide counseling to patients and their families about the benefits of identifying disease-related gene mutations and exploring innovative therapies, such as gene editing, mRNA-based treatments, and tailored immunotherapies in cases that are severe or resistant to standard treatments. Ongoing clinical monitoring is crucial in this approach to evaluate differences in treatment outcomes

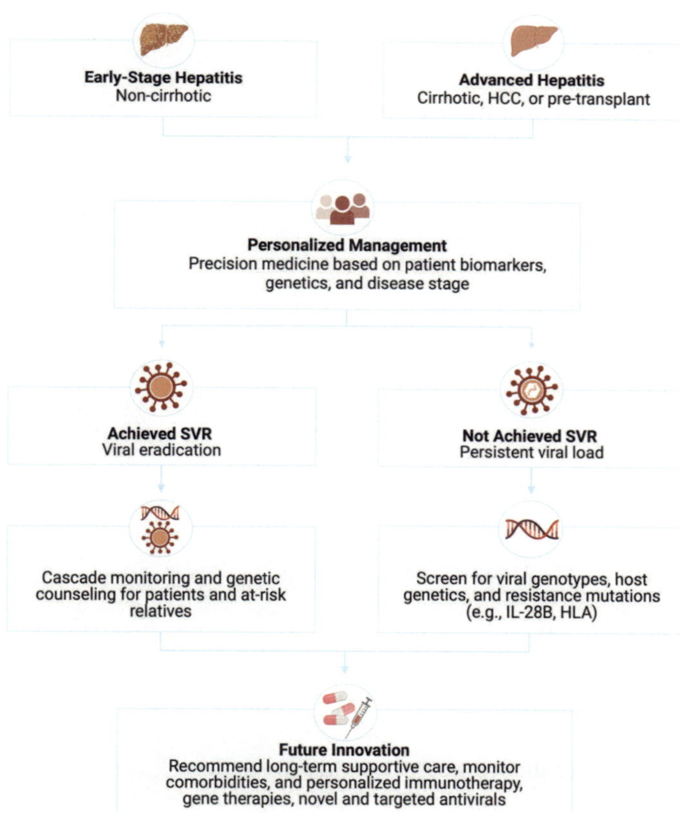

Figure 2.
Advanced clinical pathways for hepatitis patients based on personalized management Schematic outlines the advanced clinical pathways for hepatitis patients, categorized by disease stage. Personalized therapy, utilizing precision medicine and patient-specific biomarkers, is applied across groups. Abbreviations: hepatocellular carcinoma (HCC) and sustained virologic response (SVR). Generated with BioRender.com.

based on individual genetic profiles and virologic responses. By implementing this precision medicine approach, we aim to improve treatment effectiveness, safety, and long-term quality of life for hepatitis patients.

6. Conclusion

Significant advances in hepatitis management are supported by research into genetic factors enhancing treatment efficacy and minimizing resistance and toxicity. Innovations like gene editing, AI, and high-throughput sequencing have shown promising advancements in improving patient outcomes and potential cures. However, further research is essential to refine personalized treatment strategies and validate the impact of genetic variations on therapeutic responses. Future antiviral agents are anticipated to be more selective, targeting both viral replication and host factors, demonstrating the advantage of precision medicine in managing and eradicating viral hepatitis.

Conflict of interest

The authors declare no conflict of interest.

Author details

Nagham Nafiz Hendi[1,2,3]*, Asma Mahdi[3] and Randa AlYafie[2,3]

1 Faculty of Pharmacy, Middle East University, Jordan

2 Systems Biology and Immunology Department, Sidra Medicine, Doha, Qatar

3 College of Health and Life Sciences, Hamad Bin Khalifa University, Doha, Qatar

*Address all correspondence to: nhendi@sidra.org

References

[1] Alberts CJ et al. Worldwide prevalence of hepatitis B virus and hepatitis C virus among patients with cirrhosis at country, region, and global levels: A systematic review. The Lancet Gastroenterology & Hepatology. 2022;**7**(8):724-735

[2] El-Sherif O et al. Baseline factors associated with improvements in decompensated cirrhosis after direct-acting antiviral therapy for hepatitis C virus infection. Gastroenterology. 2018;**154**(8):2111-2121 e8

[3] Hindi NN, Saleh MI. Patient characteristics associated with peglyated interferon alfa-2a induced neutropenia in chronic hepatitis C patients. Clinical and Experimental Pharmacology & Physiology. 2018;**45**(7):636-642

[4] Yu X et al. Spatial transcriptomics reveals a low extent of transcriptionally active hepatitis B virus integration in patients with HBsAg loss. Gut. 2024;**73**(5):797-809

[5] Huang J et al. Hepatitis B virus pathogenesis relevant immunosignals uncovering amino acids utilization related risk factors guide artificial intelligence-based precision medicine. Frontiers in Pharmacology. 2022;**13**:1079566

[6] Jiang X, Hu J, Xie S. Construction and validation of a joint diagnosis model based on random forest and artificial intelligence network for hepatitis B-related hepatocellular carcinoma. Translational Cancer Research. 2024;**13**(2):1068-1082

[7] Sheng Z et al. Next-generation sequencing analysis of cellular response to influenza B virus infection. Viruses. 2020;**12**(4):383

[8] Woo HY et al. Comparison of mass spectrometric analysis and TRUGENE HBV genotyping for monitoring lamivudine resistance in chronic hepatitis B patients. Antiviral Therapy. 2007;**12**(1):7-13

[9] He Y et al. Identifying potential biomarkers in hepatitis B virus infection and its response to the antiviral therapy by integrated bioinformatic analysis. Journal of Cellular and Molecular Medicine. 2021;**25**(14):6558-6572

[10] Wang Z et al. Adenoviral delivery of recombinant hepatitis B virus expressing foreign antigenic epitopes for immunotherapy of persistent viral infection. Journal of Virology. 2014;**88**(5):3004-3015

[11] Kapila N et al. Fibrosing cholestatic hepatitis after kidney transplantation from HCV-viremic donors to HCV-negative recipients: A unique complication in the DAA era. American Journal of Transplantation. 2020;**20**(2):600-605

[12] World Health, O. Combating Hepatitis B and C to Reach Elimination by 2030: Advocacy Brief. Geneva: World Health Organization; 2016

[13] Angelo L et al. Pangenomic antiviral effect of REP 2139 in CRISPR/Cas9 engineered cell lines expressing hepatitis B virus surface antigen. PLoS One. 2023;**18**(11):e0293167

[14] European Association for The Study of The, L. Corrigendum to 'EASL recommendations on treatment of hepatitis C: Final update of the series' [J Hepatol 73 (2020) 1170-1218]. Journal of Hepatology. 2023;**78**(2):452

[15] European Association for the Study of the Liver. Electronic address,

e.e.e. and L. European Association for the Study of the, EASL 2017 clinical practice guidelines on the management of hepatitis B virus infection. Journal of Hepatology. 2017;**67**(2):370-398

[16] Hsu YC et al. Once-daily tenofovir disoproxil fumarate in treatment-naive Taiwanese patients with chronic hepatitis B and minimally raised alanine aminotransferase (TORCH-B): A multicentre, double-blind, placebo-controlled, parallel-group, randomised trial. The Lancet Infectious Diseases. 2021;**21**(6):823-833

[17] Zhang M et al. Effect of interferon therapy on quality of life in patients with chronic hepatitis B. Scientific Reports. 2024;**14**(1):2461

[18] Wang G et al. Potential capacity of interferon-alpha to eliminate covalently closed circular DNA (cccDNA) in hepatocytes infected with hepatitis B virus. Gut Pathogens. 2021;**13**(1):22

[19] Li J et al. Inhibition of hepatitis B virus replication by MyD88 involves accelerated degradation of pregenomic RNA and nuclear retention of pre-S/S RNAs. Journal of Virology. 2010;**84**(13):6387-6399

[20] Mertowska P et al. Immunomodulatory role of interferons in viral and bacterial infections. International Journal of Molecular Sciences. 2023;**24**(12):10115

[21] Wang D et al. Restoration of HBV-specific CD8(+) T-cell responses by sequential low-dose IL-2 treatment in non-responder patients after IFN-alpha therapy. Signal Transduction and Targeted Therapy. 2021;**6**(1):376

[22] Di Bisceglie AM et al. Recombinant interferon alfa therapy for chronic hepatitis C. A randomized, double-blind, placebo-controlled trial. The New England Journal of Medicine. 1989;**321**(22):1506-1510

[23] Wang YC et al. Predictors of response to pegylated interferon in chronic hepatitis B: A real-world hospital-based analysis. Scientific Reports. 2016;**6**:29605

[24] Saleh MI, Hindi NN. A population pharmacodynamic model characterizing neutropenia associated with pegylated interferon alpha 2-a therapy in patients with chronic hepatitis C viral infection. Naunyn-Schmiedeberg's Archives of Pharmacology. 2018;**391**(9):953-963

[25] Visco-Comandini U et al. No impact of interleukin-28B polymorphisms on spontaneous or drug-induced hepatitis delta virus clearance. Digestive and Liver Disease. 2014;**46**(4):348-352

[26] Martinez-Gomez LE et al. IL28B polymorphisms predict the response to chronic hepatitis C virus infection treatment in a Mexican population. Annals of Hepatology. 2012;**11**(6):876-881

[27] Ying SY et al. Interleukin-28B polymorphisms predict the efficacy of Peginterferon alpha in patients with chronic hepatitis B: A meta-analysis. Frontiers in Medicine (Lausanne). 2021;**8**:691365

[28] Yan ZH et al. Relationship between HLA-DR gene polymorphisms and outcomes of hepatitis B viral infections: A meta-analysis. World Journal of Gastroenterology. 2012;**18**(24):3119-3128

[29] Zhu X et al. Human leukocyte antigen class I and class II genes polymorphisms might be associated with interferon alpha therapy efficiency of chronic hepatitis B. Antiviral Research. 2011;**89**(3):189-192

[30] Li T et al. ADAR1 stimulation by IFN-alpha downregulates the expression of MAVS via RNA editing to regulate the anti-HBV response. Molecular Therapy. 2021;**29**(3):1335-1348

[31] Jiang DK et al. Genetic variation in STAT4 predicts response to interferon-alpha therapy for hepatitis B e antigen-positive chronic hepatitis B. Hepatology. 2016;**63**(4):1102-1111

[32] Boglione L et al. Extended duration of treatment with peginterferon alfa-2a in patients with chronic hepatitis B, HBeAg-negative and E genotype: A retrospective analysis. Journal of Medical Virology. 2018;**90**(6):1047-1052

[33] Chuaypen N et al. Kinetics of serum HBsAg and intrahepatic cccDNA during pegylated interferon therapy in patients with HBeAg-positive and HBeAg-negative chronic hepatitis B. Journal of Medical Virology. 2017;**89**(1):130-138

[34] Zhu YY et al. Prolonged duration of the routine pegylated-interferon alfa-2a therapy produces superior virological response in HBeAg-positive chronic hepatitis B patients: A single-center cohort study. Zhonghua Gan Zang Bing Za Zhi. 2012;**20**(10):737-741

[35] Cao ZH et al. Extended treatment with peginterferon alpha-2a in combination with lamivudine or adefovir for 96 weeks yields high rates of HBeAg and HBsAg seroconversion. Journal of Digestive Diseases. 2013;**14**(8):446-450

[36] Janssen HL et al. Pegylated interferon alfa-2b alone or in combination with lamivudine for HBeAg-positive chronic hepatitis B: A randomised trial. Lancet. 2005;**365**(9454):123-129

[37] Jiang S et al. Predictors of HBsAg seroclearance in patients with chronic HBV infection treated with pegylated interferon-alpha: A systematic review and meta-analysis. Hepatology International. 2024;**18**(3):892-903

[38] Manns MP et al. Peginterferon alfa-2b plus ribavirin compared with interferon alfa-2b plus ribavirin for initial treatment of chronic hepatitis C: A randomised trial. Lancet. 2001;**358**(9286):958-965

[39] Poynard T et al. Randomised trial of interferon alpha2b plus ribavirin for 48 weeks or for 24 weeks versus interferon alpha2b plus placebo for 48 weeks for treatment of chronic infection with hepatitis C virus. International hepatitis interventional therapy group (IHIT). Lancet. 1998;**352**(9138):1426-1432

[40] Kamar N et al. Ribavirin for hepatitis E virus infection after organ transplantation: A large European retrospective Multicenter study. Clinical Infectious Diseases. 2020;**71**(5):1204-1211

[41] European Association for the Study of the Liver. Electronic address, e.e.e. and L. European Association for the Study of the, EASL clinical practice guidelines on hepatitis E virus infection. Journal of Hepatology. 2018;**68**(6):1256-1271

[42] Nguyen DB et al. A large outbreak of hepatitis C virus infections in a Hemodialysis clinic. Infection Control and Hospital Epidemiology. 2016;**37**(2):125-133

[43] Sinclair SM et al. The ribavirin pregnancy registry: An interim analysis of potential teratogenicity at the mid-point of Enrollment. Drug Safety. 2017;**40**(12):1205-1218

[44] Rijckborst V et al. Validation of a stopping rule at week 12 using HBsAg and HBV DNA for HBeAg-negative patients treated with peginterferon

alfa-2a. Journal of Hepatology. 2012;**56**(5):1006-1011

[45] Buti M et al. Seven-year efficacy and safety of treatment with tenofovir disoproxil fumarate for chronic hepatitis B virus infection. Digestive Diseases and Sciences. 2015;**60**(5):1457-1464

[46] Jia HH et al. High prevalence of HBV lamivudine-resistant mutations in HBV/HIV Co-infected patients on antiretroviral therapy in the area with the highest prevalence of HIV/HBV Co-infection in China. Intervirology. 2018;**61**(3):123-132

[47] Lingala S et al. Long-term lamivudine therapy in chronic hepatitis B. Alimentary Pharmacology & Therapeutics. 2016;**44**(4):380-389

[48] Liaw YF et al. 2-year GLOBE trial results: Telbivudine is superior to lamivudine in patients with chronic hepatitis B. Gastroenterology. 2009;**136**(2):486-495

[49] Xu H et al. Lamivudine/telbivudine-associated neuromyopathy: Neurogenic damage, mitochondrial dysfunction and mitochondrial DNA depletion. Journal of Clinical Pathology. 2014;**67**(11):999-1005

[50] Jung TY et al. Fatal lactic acidosis in hepatitis B virus-associated decompensated cirrhosis treated with tenofovir: A case report. Medicine (Baltimore). 2017;**96**(25):e7133

[51] Ahn J et al. Entecavir safety and effectiveness in a national cohort of treatment-naive chronic hepatitis B patients in the US - the ENUMERATE study. Alimentary Pharmacology & Therapeutics. 2016;**43**(1):134-144

[52] Marcellin P et al. Ten-year efficacy and safety of tenofovir disoproxil fumarate treatment for chronic hepatitis B virus infection. Liver International. 2019;**39**(10):1868-1875

[53] Boyd A et al. Decay of ccc-DNA marks persistence of intrahepatic viral DNA synthesis under tenofovir in HIV-HBV co-infected patients. Journal of Hepatology. 2016;**65**(4):683-691

[54] Zhang X et al. Potential resistant mutations within HBV reverse transcriptase sequences in nucleos(t) ide analogues-experienced patients with hepatitis B virus infection. Scientific Reports. 2019;**9**(1):8078

[55] Fioroti CEA et al. Tenofovir-induced renal and bone toxicity: Report of two cases and literature review. Revista do Instituto de Medicina Tropical de São Paulo. 2022;**64**:e10

[56] Lampertico P et al. Switching from tenofovir disoproxil fumarate to tenofovir alafenamide in virologically suppressed patients with chronic hepatitis B: A randomised, double-blind, phase 3, multicentre non-inferiority study. The Lancet Gastroenterology & Hepatology. 2020;**5**(5):441-453

[57] Blank A et al. First-in-human application of the novel hepatitis B and hepatitis D virus entry inhibitor myrcludex B. Journal of Hepatology. 2016;**65**(3):483-489

[58] Volz T et al. The entry inhibitor Myrcludex-B efficiently blocks intrahepatic virus spreading in humanized mice previously infected with hepatitis B virus. Journal of Hepatology. 2013;**58**(5):861-867

[59] Brouwer WP et al. Adding pegylated interferon to entecavir for hepatitis B e antigen-positive chronic hepatitis B: A multicenter randomized trial (ARES study). Hepatology. 2015;**61**(5):1512-1522

[60] Hirode G et al. Off-therapy response after Nucleos(t)ide analogue withdrawal in patients with chronic hepatitis B: An international, multicenter, multiethnic cohort (RETRACT-B study). Gastroenterology. 2022;**162**(3):757-771 e4

[61] Papatheodoridis GV et al. Significance of definitions of relapse after discontinuation of oral antivirals in HBeAg-negative chronic hepatitis B. Hepatology. 2018;**68**(2):415-424

[62] Zeuzem S et al. Glecaprevir-Pibrentasvir for 8 or 12 weeks in HCV genotype 1 or 3 infection. The New England Journal of Medicine. 2018;**378**(4):354-369

[63] Quaranta MG et al. Liver function following hepatitis C virus eradication by direct acting antivirals in patients with liver cirrhosis: Data from the PITER cohort. BMC Infectious Diseases. 2021;**21**(1):413

[64] Kyuregyan KK et al. Factors influencing the prevalence of resistance-associated substitutions in NS5A protein in treatment-naive patients with chronic hepatitis C. Biomedicine. 2020;**8**(4):80

[65] Faisal N et al. Protease inhibitor-based triple therapy is highly effective for hepatitis C recurrence after liver transplant: A multicenter experience. Annals of Hepatology. 2014;**13**(5): 525-532

[66] Sulkowski M et al. Sofosbuvir and risk of estimated glomerular filtration rate decline or end-stage renal disease in patients with renal impairment. Alimentary Pharmacology & Therapeutics. 2022;**55**(9):1169-1178

[67] Naggie S et al. Ledipasvir/Sofosbuvir for 8 weeks to treat acute hepatitis C virus infections in men with human immunodeficiency virus infections: Sofosbuvir-containing regimens without interferon for treatment of acute HCV in HIV-1 infected individuals. Clinical Infectious Diseases. 2019;**69**(3):514-522

[68] Bova S et al. Access to direct-acting antivirals for hepatitis C-negative transplant recipients receiving organs from hepatitis C-viremic donors. American Journal of Health-System Pharmacy. 2022;**79**(3):173-178

[69] Forman LM et al. The association between hepatitis C infection and survival after orthotopic liver transplantation. Gastroenterology. 2002;**122**(4):889-896

[70] Crespo G et al. The efficacy of direct anti-HCV drugs improves early post-liver transplant survival and induces significant changes in waiting list composition. Journal of Hepatology. 2018;**69**(1):11-17

[71] Kapila N et al. Hepatitis C virus NAT-positive solid organ allografts transplanted into hepatitis C virus-negative recipients: A real-world experience. Hepatology. 2020;**72**(1):32-41

[72] Ting PS et al. Hepatitis C-positive donor liver transplantation for hepatitis C seronegative recipients. Transplant Infectious Disease. 2019;**21**(6):e13194

[73] Ali S et al. Improving access to the treatment of hepatitis C in low- and middle-income countries Evaluation of a patient assistance programme. International Journal of Clinical Pharmacy. 2021;**43**(4):958-968

[74] Dietz J et al. Failure on voxilaprevir, velpatasvir, sofosbuvir and efficacy of rescue therapy. Journal of Hepatology. 2021;**74**(4):801-810

[75] Reig M et al. Unexpected high rate of early tumor recurrence in patients with HCV-related HCC undergoing interferon-free therapy. Journal of Hepatology. 2016;**65**(4):719-726

[76] Cabibbo G et al. Direct-acting antivirals after successful treatment of early hepatocellular carcinoma improve survival in HCV-cirrhotic patients. Journal of Hepatology. 2019;**71**(2):265-273

[77] Gao X et al. Timing of DAA initiation after curative treatment and its relationship with the recurrence of HCV-related HCC. Journal of Hepatocellular Carcinoma. 2020;**7**:347-360

[78] Kang C, Syed YY. Bulevirtide: First approval. Drugs. 2020;**80**(15):1601-1605

[79] Petersen J, Thompson AJ, Levrero M. Aiming for cure in HBV and HDV infection. Journal of Hepatology. 2016;**65**(4):835-848

[80] de Mattos ÂZ et al. Current impact of viral hepatitis on liver cancer development: The challenge remains. World Journal of Gastroenterology. 2021;**27**(24):3556

[81] Lampertico P et al. EASL 2017 clinical practice guidelines on the management of hepatitis B virus infection. Journal of Hepatology. 2017;**67**(2):370-398

[82] Falade-Nwulia O et al. Oral direct-acting agent therapy for hepatitis C virus infection: A systematic review. Annals of Internal Medicine. 2017;**166**(9):637-648

[83] Nassal M. HBV cccDNA: Viral persistence reservoir and key obstacle for a cure of chronic hepatitis B. Gut. 2015;**64**(12):1972-1984

[84] Zai W et al. Optimized RNA interference therapeutics combined with interleukin-2 mRNA for treating hepatitis B virus infection. Signal Transduction and Targeted Therapy. 2024;**9**(1):150

[85] Zimmermann TS et al. Clinical proof of concept for a novel hepatocyte-targeting GalNAc-siRNA conjugate. Molecular Therapy. 2017;**25**(1):71-78

[86] Gane E et al. Evaluation of RNAi therapeutics VIR-2218 and ALN-HBV for chronic hepatitis B: Results from randomized clinical trials. Journal of Hepatology. 2023;**79**(4):924-932

[87] Elbadawy HM et al. Generation of combinatorial lentiviral vectors expressing multiple anti-hepatitis C virus shRNAs and their validation on a novel HCV replicon double reporter cell line. Viruses. 2020;**12**(9):1044

[88] Lee HJ et al. Targeted chromosomal duplications and inversions in the human genome using zinc finger nucleases. Genome Research. 2012;**22**(3):539-548

[89] Weber ND et al. AAV-mediated delivery of zinc finger nucleases targeting hepatitis B virus inhibits active replication. PLoS One. 2014;**9**(5):e97579

[90] Becker S, Boch J. TALE and TALEN genome editing technologies. Gene and Genome Editing. 2021;**2**:100007

[91] Smith T et al. Improved specificity and safety of anti-hepatitis B virus TALENs using obligate heterodimeric Fok I nuclease domains. Viruses. 2021;**13**(7):1344

[92] Li T et al. CRISPR/Cas9 therapeutics: Progress and prospects. Signal Transduction and Targeted Therapy. 2023;**8**(1):36

[93] Yang Y-C et al. Permanent inactivation of HBV genomes by CRISPR/Cas9-mediated non-cleavage

base editing. Molecular Therapy-Nucleic Acids. 2020;**20**:480-490

[94] Yan K et al. Inhibition of hepatitis B virus by AAV8-derived CRISPR/SaCas9 expressed from liver-specific promoters. Frontiers in Microbiology. 2021;**12**:665184

[95] Mendes BB et al. Nanodelivery of nucleic acids. Nature Reviews Methods Primers. 2022;**2**(1):24

[96] Niu C et al. Toll-like receptor 7 agonist GS-9620 induces prolonged inhibition of HBV via a type I interferon-dependent mechanism. Journal of Hepatology. 2018;**68**(5):922-931

[97] Dai L et al. Combination treatment of a TLR7 agonist RO7020531and a capsid assembly modulator RO7049389 achieved sustainable viral loadsuppression and HBsAg loss in an AAV-HBV mouse model. Journal of Hepatology. 2018;**68**:S17-S18

[98] Luk A et al. A single and multiple ascending dose study of toll-like receptor 7 agonist (RO7020531) in Chinese healthy volunteers. Clinical and Translational Science. 2020;**13**(5):985-993

[99] Yuen R et al. Ascending dose cohort study of inarigivir-a novel RIG I agonist in chronic HBV patients: Final results of the ACHIEVE trial. In: International Liver Congress 2019. Amsterdam, Netherlands: Elsevier BV; 2019. Available from: http://www.elsevier.com

[100] Gane E et al. Anti-PD-1 blockade with nivolumab with and without therapeutic vaccination for virally suppressed chronic hepatitis B: A pilot study. Journal of Hepatology. 2019;**71**(5):900-907

[101] Iannacone M, Guidotti LG. Immunobiology and pathogenesis of hepatitis B virus infection. Nature Reviews Immunology. 2022;**22**(1):19-32

[102] Koh S et al. Nonlytic lymphocytes engineered to express virus-specific T-cell receptors limit HBV infection by activating APOBEC3. Gastroenterology. 2018;**155**(1):180-193 e6

[103] Xu D-Z et al. Results of a phase III clinical trial with an HBsAg-HBIG immunogenic complex therapeutic vaccine for chronic hepatitis B patients: Experiences and findings. Journal of Hepatology. 2013;**59**(3):450-456

[104] Al Mahtab M et al. Treatment of chronic hepatitis B naïve patients with a therapeutic vaccine containing HBs and HBc antigens (a randomized, open and treatment controlled phase III clinical trial). PLoS One. 2018;**13**(3):e0201236

[105] Lok AS et al. Randomized phase II study of GS-4774 as a therapeutic vaccine in virally suppressed patients with chronic hepatitis B. Journal of Hepatology. 2016;**65**(3):509-516

[106] Zoulim F et al. Safety and immunogenicity of the therapeutic vaccine TG1050 in chronic hepatitis B patients: A phase 1b placebo-controlled trial. Human Vaccines & Immunotherapeutics. 2020;**16**(2):388-399

[107] Patra T et al. Hepatitis C virus E1 and modified E2 delivered from an mRNA vaccine induces protective immunity. npj Vaccines. 2023;**8**(1):42

[108] McGregor J et al. Virus-like particles containing the E2 core domain of hepatitis c virus generate broadly neutralizing antibodies in Guinea pigs. Journal of Virology. 2022;**96**(5):e01675-e01621

[109] Mekonnen ZA et al. Enhanced T cell responses induced by a necrotic

dendritic cell vaccine, expressing HCV NS3. Frontiers in Microbiology. 2020;**11**:559105

[110] Fanning GC et al. Therapeutic strategies for hepatitis B virus infection: Towards a cure. Nature Reviews Drug Discovery. 2019;**18**(11):827-844

[111] Boni C et al. Combined GS-4774 and tenofovir therapy can improve HBV-specific T-cell responses in patients with chronic hepatitis. Gastroenterology. 2019;**157**(1):227-241 e7

[112] De Mot L et al. Transcriptional profiles of adjuvanted hepatitis B vaccines display variable interindividual homogeneity but a shared core signature. Science Translational Medicine. 2020;**12**(569):eaay8618

[113] Yang S et al. Factors influencing immunologic response to hepatitis B vaccine in adults. Scientific Reports. 2016;**6**(1):27251

[114] Rajoriya N et al. How viral genetic variants and genotypes influence disease and treatment outcome of chronic hepatitis B. Time for an individualised approach? Journal of Hepatology. 2017;**67**(6):1281-1297

[115] Bellavite P. Causality assessment of adverse events following immunization: The problem of multifactorial pathology. F1000Research. 2020;**9**:170

[116] Zhu C et al. Nanoparticle-driven biosensors for diagnosis of viral hepatitis. TrAC Trends in Analytical Chemistry. 2024;**180**:117985

[117] Prasidthrathsint K, Stapleton JT. Laboratory diagnosis and monitoring of viral hepatitis. Gastroenterology Clinics of North America. 2019;**48**(2):259-279

[118] Dembele B et al. Evaluation of four rapid tests for detection of hepatitis B surface antigen in Ivory Coast. Journal of Immunology Research. 2020;**2020**:6315718

[119] Chevaliez S et al. Performance of rapid diagnostic tests for hepatitis B surface antigen detection in serum or plasma. Diagnostic Microbiology and Infectious Disease. 2021;**100**(2):115353

[120] Quinones-Mateu ME et al. Deep sequencing: Becoming a critical tool in clinical virology. Journal of Clinical Virology. 2014;**61**(1):9-19

[121] Solmone M et al. Use of massively parallel ultradeep pyrosequencing to characterize the genetic diversity of hepatitis B virus in drug-resistant and drug-naive patients and to detect minor variants in reverse transcriptase and hepatitis B S antigen. Journal of Virology. 2009;**83**(4):1718-1726

[122] Garcia-Garcia S et al. Next-generation sequencing for the diagnosis of hepatitis B: Current status and future prospects. Expert Review of Molecular Diagnostics. 2021;**21**(4):381-396

[123] Palacios G et al. A new arenavirus in a cluster of fatal transplant-associated diseases. The New England Journal of Medicine. 2008;**358**(10):991-998

[124] Quick J et al. Multiplex PCR method for MinION and Illumina sequencing of Zika and other virus genomes directly from clinical samples. Nature Protocols. 2017;**12**(6):1261-1276

[125] Towner JS et al. Newly discovered ebola virus associated with hemorrhagic fever outbreak in Uganda. PLoS Pathogens. 2008;**4**(11):e1000212

[126] Ge X et al. Metagenomic analysis of viruses from bat fecal samples reveals many novel viruses in insectivorous bats in China. Journal of Virology. 2012;**86**(8):4620-4630

[127] Yozwiak NL et al. Virus identification in unknown tropical febrile illness cases using deep sequencing. PLoS Neglected Tropical Diseases. 2012;**6**(2):e1485

[128] Dopico E et al. Genotyping hepatitis B virus by next-generation sequencing: Detection of mixed infections and analysis of sequence conservation. International Journal of Molecular Sciences. 2024;**25**(10):5481

[129] Botkin JR, Rothwell E. Whole genome sequencing and newborn screening. Current Genetic Medicine Reports. 2016;**4**(1):1-6

[130] Li W et al. Multiple immune defects in two patients with novel DOCK2 mutations result in recurrent multiple infection including live attenuated virus vaccine. Journal of Clinical Immunology. 2023;**43**(6):1193-1207

[131] Georges N, Nagham Nafiz H. Pharmacogenomics of cardiovascular diseases: The path to precision therapy. In: Madhu K, Anupam M, Amol P, editors. Pharmacogenomics and Pharmacogenetics in Drug Therapy. IntechOpen: Rijeka; 2023. p. Ch. 5

[132] Swen JJ et al. Pharmacogenetic information in clinical guidelines: The European perspective. Clinical Pharmacology and Therapeutics. 2018;**103**(5):795-801

[133] Wang L et al. Implementation of preemptive DNA sequence-based pharmacogenomics testing across a large academic medical center: The Mayo-Baylor RIGHT 10K study. Genetics in Medicine. 2022;**24**(5):1062-1072

[134] Irham LM et al. The use of genomic variants to drive drug repurposing for chronic hepatitis B. Biochemistry and Biophysics Reports. 2022;**31**:101307

[135] Akcay IM et al. Host genetic factors affecting hepatitis B infection outcomes: Insights from genome-wide association studies. World Journal of Gastroenterology. 2018;**24**(30):3347-3360

[136] Motsinger-Reif AA et al. Genome-wide association studies in pharmacogenomics: Successes and lessons. Pharmacogenetics and Genomics. 2013;**23**(8):383-394

[137] Popejoy AB. Diversity in precision medicine and pharmacogenetics: Methodological and conceptual considerations for broadening participation. Pharmacogenomics and Personalized Medicine. 2019;**12**:257-271

[138] Yang TH et al. Genetic susceptibility to hepatocellular carcinoma in patients with chronic hepatitis virus infection. Viruses. 2023;**15**(2):559

[139] Kamatani Y et al. A genome-wide association study identifies variants in the HLA-DP locus associated with chronic hepatitis B in Asians. Nature Genetics. 2009;**41**(5):591-595

[140] Ou G, Liu X, Jiang Y. HLA-DPB1 alleles in hepatitis B vaccine response: A meta-analysis. Medicine (Baltimore). 2021;**100**(14):e24904

[141] Wu TW et al. Common genetic variants of response to hepatitis B vaccines correlate with risks of chronic infection of hepatitis B virus: A community-based case-control study. International Journal of Molecular Sciences. 2023;**24**(11):9741

[142] Qiu B et al. Advances in the genome-wide association study of chronic hepatitis B susceptibility in Asian population. European Journal of Medical Research. 2017;**22**(1):55

[143] Trinks J et al. Role of HLA-DP and HLA-DQ on the clearance of hepatitis B virus and the risk of chronic infection in a multiethnic population. Liver International. 2017;**37**(10):1476-1487

[144] Talangescu A et al. Molecular analysis of HLA genes in Romanian patients with chronic hepatitis B virus infection. Current Issues in Molecular Biology. 2024;**46**(2):1064-1077

[145] Li H et al. Single nucleotide polymorphisms in ZNF208 are associated with increased risk for HBV in Chinese people. Oncotarget. 2017;**8**(68):112451-112459

[146] Miri HH et al. Correlation between IL-28 polymorphism and spontaneous clearance in HCV patients: Systematic review and meta-analysis. Archives of Virology. 2021;**166**(9):2469-2478

[147] Ge D et al. Genetic variation in IL28B predicts hepatitis C treatment-induced viral clearance. Nature. 2009;**461**(7262):399-401

[148] Matsuura K, Watanabe T, Tanaka Y. Role of IL28B for chronic hepatitis C treatment toward personalized medicine. Journal of Gastroenterology and Hepatology. 2014;**29**(2):241-249

[149] Hayes CN et al. Genetics of IL28B and HCV–response to infection and treatment. Nature Reviews. Gastroenterology & Hepatology. 2012;**9**(7):406-417

[150] Bhushan A et al. Confounding by single nucleotide polymorphism rs117648444 (P70S) affects the Association of Interferon Lambda Locus Variants with response to interferon-alpha-ribavirin therapy in patients with chronic genotype 3 hepatitis C virus infection. Journal of Interferon & Cytokine Research. 2017;**37**(8):369-382

[151] Ito K et al. The rs8099917 polymorphism, when determined by a suitable genotyping method, is a better predictor for response to pegylated alpha interferon/ribavirin therapy in Japanese patients than other single nucleotide polymorphisms associated with interleukin-28B. Journal of Clinical Microbiology. 2011;**49**(5):1853-1860

[152] Riva E et al. Hepatitis C virus and interferon type III (interferon-lambda3/interleukin-28B and interferon-lambda4): Genetic basis of susceptibility to infection and response to antiviral treatment. Clinical Microbiology and Infection. 2014;**20**(12):1237-1245

[153] Ibrahim MK et al. The impact of genetic variations in sofosbuvir metabolizing enzymes and innate immunity mediators on treatment outcome in HCV-infected patients. Microbial Pathogenesis. 2022;**162**:105311

[154] Loucks CM et al. Patient-specific genetic factors predict treatment failure in sofosbuvir-treated patients with chronic hepatitis C. Liver International. 2022;**42**(4):796-808

[155] Mohamed Abdelnajid D et al. Prediction of response to sofosbuvir-based therapy using serum interleukin-12 and single nucleotide polymorphism of the interleukin 28B gene as predictive factors in HCV positive genotype-4 patients. Medicine (Baltimore). 2023;**102**(28):e34125

[156] Suppiah V et al. IL28B is associated with response to chronic hepatitis C interferon-alpha and ribavirin therapy. Nature Genetics. 2009;**41**(10):1100-1104

[157] Tanaka Y et al. Genome-wide association of IL28B with response to pegylated interferon-alpha and ribavirin therapy for chronic hepatitis C. Nature Genetics. 2009;**41**(10):1105-1109

[158] Heim MH, Bochud PY, George J. Host - hepatitis C viral interactions: The role of genetics. Journal of Hepatology. 2016;**65**(1 Suppl.):S22-S32

[159] Asthana M et al. Role of interleukin 28B polymorphisms in response to interferon based therapy for hepatitis C virus clearance. Current Drug Metabolism. 2018;**19**(3):215-223

[160] Ansari MA et al. Interferon lambda 4 impacts the genetic diversity of hepatitis C virus. eLife. 2019;**8**:e42463

[161] Ferreira J et al. Role of inflammatory/immune response and cytokine polymorphisms in the severity of chronic hepatitis C (CHC) before and after direct acting antiviral (DAAs) treatment. International journal of molecular sciences. 2023;**24**(2):1380

[162] Zaki SM et al. Interleukin 28B polymorphism as a predictor of sustained virological response to sofosbuvir-based therapy for hepatitis C virus patients. Tropical Medicine and Infectious Disease. 2022;**7**(9):230

[163] Echeverria N et al. IL28B gene polymorphism rs12979860, but not rs8099917, contributes to the occurrence of chronic HCV infection in Uruguayan patients. Virology Journal. 2018;**15**(1):40

[164] Domagalski K et al. The impact of IL28B genotype and liver fibrosis on the hepatic expression of IP10, IFI27, ISG15, and MX1 and their association with treatment outcomes in patients with chronic hepatitis C. PLoS One. 2015;**10**(6):e0130899

[165] McCarthy JJ et al. Replicated association between an IL28B gene variant and a sustained response to pegylated interferon and ribavirin. Gastroenterology. 2010;**138**(7):2307-2314

[166] Gao Y, Nepal N, Jin SZ. Toll-like receptors and hepatitis C virus infection. Hepatobiliary & Pancreatic Diseases International. 2021;**20**(6):521-529

[167] Hamdy S et al. Association of Toll-like receptor 3 and toll-like receptor 9 single-nucleotide polymorphisms with hepatitis C virus persistence among Egyptians. Archives of Virology. 2018;**163**(9):2433-2442

[168] Chen Q et al. Interferon lambda 4 impairs hepatitis C viral antigen presentation and attenuates T cell responses. Nature Communications. 2021;**12**(1):4882

[169] Jefferies CA. Regulating IRFs in IFN driven disease. Frontiers in Immunology. 2019;**10**:325

[170] Talaat RM et al. Genetic polymorphism in toll-like receptor 3 and interferon regulatory factor 3 in hepatitis C virus-infected patients: Correlation with liver cirrhosis. Viral Immunology. 2022;**35**(9):609-615

[171] Badami E et al. Hepatocellular carcinoma, hepatitis C virus infection and miRNA involvement: Perspectives for new therapeutic approaches. World Journal of Gastroenterology. 2022;**28**(22):2417-2428

[172] Qian X et al. Hepatitis C virus infection cycle-specific MicroRNA profiling reveals stage-specific miR-4423-3p targets RIG-I to facilitate infection. Frontiers in Cellular and Infection Microbiology. 2022;**12**:851917

[173] Howard HC et al. Whole-genome sequencing in newborn screening? A statement on the continued importance of targeted approaches in newborn screening programmes. European Journal of Human Genetics. 2015;**23**(12):1593-1600

[174] Bienfait K et al. Current challenges and opportunities for pharmacogenomics: Perspective of the industry pharmacogenomics working group (I-PWG). Human Genetics. 2022;**141**(6):1165-1173

[175] Trauger SA, Junker T, Siuzdak G. Investigating viral proteins and intact viruses with mass spectrometry. In: Schalley C, editor. Modern Mass Spectrometry. Berlin, Germany: Springer; 2003

[176] Worner TP et al. Mass spectrometry-based structural virology. Analytical Chemistry. 2021;**93**(1):620-640

[177] Mohamed EI et al. Electronic nose versus quadrupole mass spectrometry for identifying viral hepatitis C patients. Journal of Viral Hepatitis. 2022;**29**(2):147-155

[178] Albalat A et al. Classical MALDI-MS versus CE-based ESI-MS proteomic profiling in urine for clinical applications. Bioanalysis. 2014;**6**(2):247-266

[179] Milewska A et al. Mass spectrometry in Virological sciences. Mass Spectrometry Reviews. 2020;**39**(5-6):499-522

[180] Piao J et al. Simultaneous detection and identification of enteric viruses by PCR-mass assay. PLoS One. 2012;**7**(8):e42251

[181] Hong SP et al. Detection of hepatitis B virus YMDD variants using mass spectrometric analysis of oligonucleotide fragments. Journal of Hepatology. 2004;**40**(5):837-844

[182] Zai W et al. Long-term hepatitis B virus infection induces cytopathic effects in primary human hepatocytes, and can Be partially reversed by antiviral therapy. Microbiology Spectrum. 2022;**10**(1):e0132821

[183] Murphy CM et al. Hepatitis B virus X protein promotes degradation of SMC5/6 to enhance HBV replication. Cell Reports. 2016;**16**(11):2846-2854

[184] Pan HY et al. LC/MS-based global metabolomic identification of serum biomarkers differentiating hepatocellular carcinoma from chronic hepatitis B and liver cirrhosis. ACS Omega. 2021;**6**(2):1160-1170

[185] Hu J et al. Hexosamine biosynthetic pathway promotes the antiviral activity of SAMHD1 by enhancing O-GlcNAc transferase-mediated protein O-GlcNAcylation. Theranostics. 2021;**11**(2):805-823

[186] Simillion C et al. Robust regression analysis of GCMS data reveals differential rewiring of metabolic networks in hepatitis B and C patients. Metabolites. 2017;**7**(4):51

[187] Liu Z et al. Determination of candidate metabolite biomarkers associated with recurrence of HCV-related hepatocellular carcinoma. Oncotarget. 2018;**9**(5):6245-6258

[188] Su TH, Wu CH, Kao JH. Artificial intelligence in precision medicine in hepatology. Journal of Gastroenterology and Hepatology. 2021;**36**(3):569-580

[189] Fei L et al. CRISPR/Cas9 system with dual gRNAs Synergically inhibit hepatitis B virus replication. Discovery Medicine. 2024;**36**(185):1169-1179

[190] Zeng H et al. High-throughput sequencing-based analysis of gene expression of hepatitis B virus infection-associated human hepatocellular carcinoma. Oncology Letters. 2020;**20**(4):18

[191] Ashouri S et al. Genome-wide association study for chronic hepatitis B infection in the Thai population. Frontiers in Genetics. 2022;**13**:887121

[192] Wallis C et al. Hepatitis C virus point-of-care RNA testing: Experience from screening an entire high-security Australian prison population over 3 days. Australian and New Zealand Journal of Public Health. 2023;**47**(5):100083